W9-ACF-559

Study Guide for Leifer

Introduction to Maternity and Pediatric Nursing

7th Edition

Emily Slone McKinney, MSN, RN, C
Baylor Healthcare System
Women and Children's Services
Dallas, Texas

ELSEVIER
SAUNDERS

ELSEVIER

SAUNDERS

3251 Riverport Lane
St. Louis, Missouri 63043

Senior Vice President and General Manager, Content: Loren Wilson
Content Strategist: Nancy O'Brien
Associate Content Development Specialist: Jacqueline Kiley
Publishing Services Manager: Jeff Patterson
Senior Project Manager: Jeanne Genz
Senior Book Designer: Karen Pauls
Composition Services: Lisa Hernandez

Printed in the United States of America

Last digit is the print number: 9 8 7 6 5 4 3 2

Preface

Understanding fundamental concepts and principles of nursing will prepare you for patient care experiences. By mastering the content of your *Introduction to Maternity and Pediatric Nursing* textbook, you will have the necessary knowledge and skills for practice. This Study Guide was created to help you achieve the objectives of each chapter in the textbook, establish a solid base of knowledge, and evaluate your understanding of this critical information.

Matching and completion **Learning Activities** help reinforce basic factual knowledge from the textbook that underlies nursing care. Other exercises ask you to list or describe text information to encourage reading comprehension and written expression of what is learned. Labeling of illustrations is included to help you understand anatomy, as appropriate.

Each chapter contains multiple choice **Review Questions** that ask for appropriate nursing actions, what the nurse should expect in terms of medical orders or usual care of the patient, and potential complications, as well as items that review basic factual information from the chapter.

Some chapters include **Crossword Puzzles** to further test comprehension of terms and concepts.

To promote higher-level learning, **Thinking Critically** activities ask you to apply knowledge or draw conclusions based on material not directly answered in the textbook. **Case Studies** and **Applying Knowledge** activities provide ideas for applying factual content to patient care.

An answer key for the Learning Activities, Review Questions, Crossword Puzzles, and selected Thinking Critically activities and Case Studies is available on the Student Evolve website.

To maximize the benefits of this Study Guide and prepare for the learning activities:

1. Carefully read the textbook chapter and highlight, note, or outline important information.
2. Review the Key Points, access the Additional Learning Resources, and complete the Review Questions for the NCLEX® Examination at the end of each textbook chapter.
3. Complete the Study Guide exercises to the best of your ability.
4. Time and pace yourself during the completion of each exercise. You should spend approximately 1 minute for each multiple choice, true/false, and matching question, and approximately 2 minutes for completion activities or short answer questions.
5. After completing an exercise, refer to the textbook page references as needed. You can then repeat any exercises for additional practice and review. A complete answer key can be found on the Student Evolve website.

STUDY HINTS FOR ALL STUDENTS

- *Ask questions!* There are no bad questions. If you do not know something or are not sure, you need to find out. Other people may be wondering the same thing but may be too shy to ask. The answer could mean life or death to your patient, which certainly is more important than feeling embarrassed about asking a question.
- *Make use of chapter objectives.* At the beginning of each chapter in the textbook are objectives that you should have mastered when you finish studying that chapter. Write these objectives in your notebook, leaving a blank space after each. Fill in the answers as you find them while reading the chapter. Review to make sure your answers are correct and complete, and use these answers when you study for tests. This should also be done for separate course objectives that your instructor has listed in your class syllabus.
- *Locate and understand key terms.* At the beginning of each chapter in the textbook are key terms that you will encounter as you read the chapter. Page numbers are provided for easy reference and review, and the key terms are in bold, blue font the first time they appear in the chapter. Phonetic pronunciations are provided for terms that might be difficult to pronounce.
- *Review Key Points.* Use the Key Points at the end of each chapter in the textbook to help you review for exams.
- *Get the most from your textbook.* When reading each chapter in the textbook, look at the subject headings to learn what each section is about. Read first for the general meaning, then reread parts you did not understand. It may help to read those parts aloud. Carefully read the information given in each table and study each figure and its caption.
- *Follow up on difficult concepts.* While studying, put difficult concepts into your own words to see if you understand them. Check this understanding with another student or the instructor. Write these in your notebook.
- *Take useful notes.* When taking lecture notes in class, leave a large margin on the left side of each notebook page and write only on right-hand pages, leaving all left-hand pages blank. Look over your lecture notes soon after

each class, while your memory is fresh. Fill in missing words, complete sentences and ideas, and underline key phrases, definitions, and concepts. At the top of each page, write the topic of that page. In the left margin, write the key word for that part of your notes. On the opposite left-hand page, write a summary or outline that combines material from both the textbook and the lecture. These can be your study notes for review.

- *Join or form a study group.* Form a study group with some other students so you can help one another. Practice speaking and reading aloud, ask questions about material you are not sure about, and work together to find answers.

- *Improve your study skills.* Good study skills are essential for achieving your goals in nursing. Time management, efficient use of study time, and a consistent approach to studying are all beneficial. There are various study methods for reading a textbook and for taking class notes. Some methods that have proven helpful can be found in *Saunders Student Nurse Planner: A Guide to Success in Nursing School* by Susan C. deWit. This book contains helpful information on test-taking and preparing for clinical experiences. It includes an example of a "time map" for planning study time and a blank form that you can use to formulate a personal time map.

ADDITIONAL STUDY HINTS FOR STUDENTS WHO USE ENGLISH AS A SECOND LANGUAGE (ESL)

- *Find a first-language buddy.* ESL students should find a first-language buddy—another student who is a native speaker of English and is willing to answer questions about word meanings, pronunciations, and culture. Maybe your buddy would like to learn about your language and culture. This could help in his or her nursing experience as well.

- *Expand your vocabulary.* If you find a nontechnical word you do not know (e.g., *drowsy*), try to guess its meaning from the sentence (e.g., *With electrolyte imbalance, the patient may feel fatigued and drowsy*). If you are not sure of the meaning, or if it seems particularly important, look it up in the dictionary.

- *Keep a vocabulary notebook.* Keep a small alphabetized notebook or address book in which you can write down new nontechnical words you read or hear along with their meanings and pronunciations. Write each word under its initial letter so you can find it easily, as in a dictionary. For words you do not know or for words that have a different meaning in nursing, write down how they are used and sound. Look up their meanings in a dictionary or ask your instructor or first-language buddy. Then write the different meanings or usages that you have found in your book, including the nursing meaning. Continue to add new words as you discover them. For example:
  - *Primary—Of most importance; main (e.g., the primary problem or disease); The first one; elementary (e.g., primary school)*
  - *Secondary—Of less importance; resulting from another problem or disease (e.g., a secondary symptom); The second one (e.g., secondary school ["high school" in the United States])*

Illustration Credits

Figures 2-1, 2-2, 2-3, 2-4: From Herlihy, B., & Maebius, N.K. (2011). *The human body in health and illness* (4th ed.). Philadelphia: Saunders.

Figure 2-5: Modified from *Stedman's illustrated medical dictionary* (25th ed.). Baltimore: Williams & Wilkins.

Figure 2-6: From Seidel, H.M., et al. (2011). *Mosby's guide to physical examination* (7th ed.). St. Louis: Mosby.

Figure 3-1: From McKinney, E.S., et al. (2009). *Maternal-child nursing* (5th ed.). St. Louis: Saunders.

Figure 23-1: From Hockenberry, M., Wilson, D., Winkelstein, M.L., & Kline, N.E. (2011). *Wong's nursing care of infants and children* (9th ed.). St. Louis: Mosby.

Figure 24-1: From Swisher, L., Thibodeau, G.A., & Patton, K.T. (2009). *Study guide for the human body in health and disease* (5th ed.). St. Louis: Mosby.

Figure 29-1: Art overlay courtesy Observatory Group, Cincinnati, Ohio.

The Past, Present, and Future

chapter

1

Answer Key: A complete answer key can be found on the Student Evolve website.

LEARNING ACTIVITIES

1. Match the terms in the left column with their definitions on the right (a–k).

_____ Advanced-practice nurse *(10)*

_____ Clinical pathways *(12)*

_____ Diagnosis-related groups (DRGs) *(8)*

_____ Empowerment *(2)*

_____ Evidence-based practice *(14)*

_____ Family-centered care *(2)*

_____ Full inclusion *(10)*

_____ Health maintenance organization (HMO) *(9)*

_____ Managed care *(9)*

_____ Preferred provider organization (PPO) *(9)*

_____ Variance *(12)*

a. The difference between the expected outcome and the outcome achieved

b. Recognizing the strength and integrity of the family as the core of planning and implementing health care

c. A registered nurse with an advanced degree who specializes in a clinical area of nursing such as obstetrics or pediatrics and may conduct research in his or her specialty

d. Expansion of mainstreaming process to integrate a physically or mentally challenged child into society

e. A system used by government-financed programs that determines payment for a person's hospital stay based on the diagnosis

f. A health organization that contracts with providers for services at a discount for its members

g. A health care delivery system that contracts with providers to provide services at a fixed capitated fee each month

h. An organization that offers health services for a fixed premium

i. Research-based guidelines for expected progress within a timeline

j. Providing the means by which families accept and maintain control over their members' health care

k. Nursing practice based on the most current data available through valid research

2. List three health care professionals who deliver babies. *(2)*

   a. _____

   b. _____

   c. _____

3. Match the names in the left column with their contributions toward improvement of maternal, newborn, and pediatric care on the right (a–j).

_____ Samuel Bard *(3)*	a. Associated unwashed hands of medical students following dissection of cadavers and puerperal fever among postpartum women
_____ Karl Credé *(2)*	b. Determined that puerperal fever was caused by bacteria that could be spread by people and objects
_____ Abraham Jacobi *(2)*	
_____ Oliver Wendell Holmes *(3)*	c. Helped establish the Children's Bureau, leading to birth registration and school lunch programs
_____ Joseph Lister *(2)*	
_____ Louis Pasteur *(2)*	d. Developed a treatment to prevent infant blindness caused by gonorrhea
_____ Margaret Sanger *(16)*	e. Wrote a paper about the contagiousness of puerperal fever, thus initiating the germ theory of disease
_____ Ignaz Semmelweis *(2)*	
_____ Soranus *(2)*	f. Wrote the first American textbook on obstetrics for midwives
_____ Lillian Wald *(4)*	g. Applied antiseptic principles to surgical practice
	h. Introduced podalic version to deliver the second twin
	i. Established pediatric nursing as a medical specialty
	j. Provided care for poor pregnant women, which was the seed for development of today's Planned Parenthood programs

4. List three professional organizations concerned with maternity nursing. *(3)*

   a. _____

   b. _____

   c. _____

5. Describe how each listed governmental program influences maternity and pediatric care.

   a. Sheppard-Towner Act: *(3)*_____

   _____

   _____

b. Title V Amendment of the Social Security Act: *(3)* _____

_____

_____

c. Title XIX of the Medicaid program: *(4)* _____

_____

_____

d. Head Start program: *(3)* _____

_____

_____

e. National Center for Family Planning: *(3)* _____

_____

_____

f. Women, Infants, and Children (WIC) Program: *(3)* _____

_____

_____

g. Family and Medical Leave Act (FMLA): *(3)* _____

_____

_____

h. Fair Labor Standards Act: *(3)* _____

_____

_____

i. Education for All Handicapped Children Act: *(3)* _____

_____

_____

j. Missing Children's Act: *(3)* _____

_____

_____

6. How has the inpatient stay for birth changed recently? What are the numbers of babies born vaginally and the numbers born by cesarean? What implication do you believe these changes have for nurses? *(3)*

_____

_____

7. How have consumers changed practices in maternity care? *(6)* _____

_____

_____

8. Give examples of how technology and development of medical specialties affects the care of infants and children. *(8)*

_____

_____

_____

_____

9. How have advances in technology contributed to the growing population of chronically ill children? *(8)*

_____

_____

10. List the six steps of the nursing process. *(11)*

   a. _____

   b. _____

   c. _____

   d. _____

   e. _____

   f. _____

11. What is the place of the *Nursing Interventions Classification (NIC)* and *Nursing Outcome Criteria (NOC)* in patient care and reimbursement for nursing services? *(12, 14)*

_____

_____

_____

_____

12. Explain the meaning and use of critical thinking in nursing. *(11; Box 1-8)* _____

_____

_____

_____

_____

13. What is *Healthy People 2010/2020?* (16)_____

_____

_____

_____

REVIEW QUESTIONS

1. The most important nursing action to prevent infection in any patient is to: *(2)*
   1. use disposable equipment.
   2. consistently perform hand hygiene.
   3. limit visitors to family members.
   4. wear hospital-laundered clothes.

2. To best improve the care of a pregnant woman from a different cultural group, the nurse should: *(6-7, Nursing Care Plan 1-1)*
   1. identify the woman's expectations about pregnancy and birth.
   2. observe the woman and her family as they interact.
   3. learn about members of different local cultural groups.
   4. encourage the woman to adopt local childbearing practices.

3. One of the most effective ways nurses may use statistics is to: *(12)*
   1. determine daily staffing to maintain the best patient care.
   2. predict the hospital census for the following year.
   3. evaluate the outcomes of prenatal care provided.
   4. compute the number of women who conceive each year.

4. Choose the best description of certified nurse-midwife (CNM) qualifications. *(6)*
   1. Gives limited care to women after normal childbirth
   2. Assists in the prenatal care of high-risk women
   3. Primarily provides care to low-income women
   4. Attends uncomplicated births of low-risk women

5. The nursing process is best described as a method to: *(11)*
   1. identify patients who have an increased risk for medical complications.
   2. reduce the incidence of complications for expectant mothers and infants.
   3. identify and solve patient problems with individualized nursing care.
   4. promote breastfeeding in groups that do not usually nurse infants.

6. Choose the best description for a variance in a clinical pathway. *(12)*
   1. The patient did not cooperate with the recommended therapy.
   2. An achieved patient outcome differs from the expected outcome.
   3. Patient care is individualized, appropriate to a specific person.
   4. Reimbursement will be curtailed because of a complication.

APPLYING KNOWLEDGE

1. What is the typical hospital stay for the following patients at your clinical site?
   a. A woman who has an uncomplicated vaginal birth
   b. A woman who has an uncomplicated cesarean birth

2. Do insurance companies or HMOs offer home visits to women who had uncomplicated births? Ask several nurses how they manage their care to accommodate short postpartum hospital stays.

3. Talk with a father who was present at the birth of his child.
    a. How did the experience affect him?
    b. If he has more than one child and was not present at all of the births, does he perceive any differences in how he feels toward his children based on whether he was present at their births? Did active military service cause him to miss the births?

4. When you are in the clinical area, care for a childbearing family from a cultural group other than your own.
    a. Use the assessment questions listed under Cultural Considerations on p. 6 in your text to better understand the family's views toward birth.
    b. When you are in the clinical area, observe how the family is involved in the birth process.

5. Talk to new grandparents about how birth has changed since their children were born. Use the following questions as a springboard for discussion or answer them individually.
    a. Were you involved in the birth of your children?
    b. What pain relief was available where you gave birth?
    c. How do you feel about the involvement of fathers in childbirth?
    d. How do cultural influences seem to affect women and their families when birth occurs? Do you see differences between new immigrant families and those who have been in our country for more than one generation?
    e. Do you think siblings of the new baby should be involved during or after birth? If so, in what way?

6. Ask the birth facility in your clinical area what types of statistical data they gather and what is done with that data. Use www.cdc.gov/nchs to locate the most recent information about number of births, term births, preterm births, and low–birth-weight infants. What were the percentages of cesarean births and vaginal births during the most recent year at your clinical facility?

7. Does your clinical facility use a method of electronic documentation? What security measures ensure privacy of a patient's data? What arrangements does the facility have if the computer system is down? How do you chart your assessments and nursing actions when in your clinical area?

8. Describe how you use critical thinking to solve problems or meet needs in daily nonnursing aspects of your life.

Human Reproductive Anatomy and Physiology

Answer Key: A complete answer key can be found on the Student Evolve website.

LEARNING ACTIVITIES

1. _____ is the time when reproductive systems mature and become capable of reproduction. *(20)*

2. a. Hormonal changes of puberty in boys begin between the ages of _____ and _____ years. *(20)*

   b. The first outward male changes of puberty are growth of the _____ and _____. *(20)*

3. a. The first outward female change of puberty is _____ _____. *(21)*

   b. The first menstrual period usually occurs _____ years after this initial change. *(21)*

4. Describe secondary sexual characteristics in boys and girls. *(21-22)*

   a. Boys: _____

   _____

   b. Girls: _____

   _____

5. Match the terms in the left column with their definitions on the right (a–h).

   _____ Androgens *(21)*

   _____ Penis *(21)*

   _____ Scrotum *(21)*

   _____ Semen *(22)*

   _____ Spermatogenesis *(21)*

   _____ Spermatozoa *(21)*

   _____ Testes *(21)*

   _____ Testosterone *(21)*

   a. Organs that produce spermatozoa and male sex hormones
   b. Seminal plasma plus sperm
   c. Male sex hormones
   d. Primary male hormone
   e. Male germ (reproductive) cells
   f. Male organ for urination and sexual intercourse
   g. Production of spermatozoa
   h. Skin sac that suspends testes away from the body

6. Label the structures of the male reproductive system on the figure below. *(21)*

   a. Anus
   b. Bulbourethral gland
   c. Ejaculatory duct
   d. Epididymis
   e. Foreskin of penis
   f. Glans penis
   g. Penis
   h. Prostate gland
   i. Scrotum
   j. Seminal vesicle
   k. Testis
   l. Urethra
   m. Urinary bladder
   n. Vas deferens

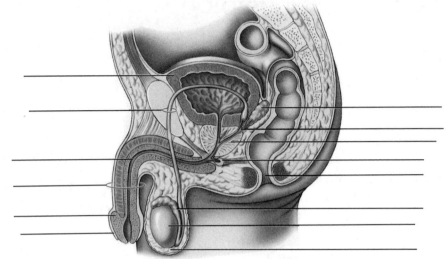

7. a. Spermatozoa are produced in the _____ _____ of the testes. *(22)*

   b. Testosterone is produced in the _____ _____ of the testes. *(22)*

8. Describe six effects of testosterone. *(22)*

   a. _____

   b. _____

   c. _____

   d. _____

   e. _____

   f. _____

9. Label the structures of the external female genitalia on the figure below. *(23)*

a. Anus
b. Clitoris
c. Labia majora
d. Labia minora
e. Mons pubis
f. Opening for vestibular glands
g. Perineum
h. Urethra
i. Vagina

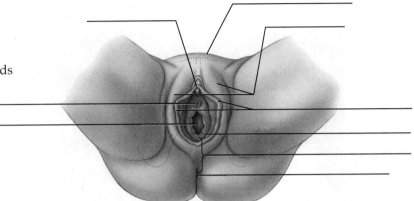

10. Match each female reproductive organ with its function or functions (a–r). More than one letter may be used for some organs.

_____ Bartholin's glands (vulvovaginal glands) *(23, 29)*

_____ Cervical mucosal lining *(24)*

_____ Cervix *(24)*

_____ Clitoris *(22)*

_____ Endometrium *(24)*

_____ Fallopian tubes *(24-25; Fig. 2-3 and 2-4)*

_____ Myometrium *(24)*

_____ Ovaries *(25)*

_____ Rugae *(23)*

_____ Skene's ducts (paraurethral ducts) *(22)*

_____ Urethral meatus *(22)*

_____ Uterus *(23-24)*

_____ Vagina *(23)*

_____ Vaginal introitus *(22)*

a. Location for implantation of the fertilized ovum and growth of fetus
b. Female organ of sexual intercourse
c. Uterine layer that responds to hormone changes during the menstrual cycle
d. Sensitive erectile body that gives erotic sensations when stimulated
e. Passage for menstrual flow and fetus
f. Folds or ridges of the vaginal mucous membrane
g. Produce vaginal lubrication during sexual arousal
h. Uterine layer in which fertilized ovum implants
i. Site of fertilization and early embryonic development
j. Produce ova (female germ cells) and female hormones
k. Muscular uterine layer to expel fetus at birth
l. Provides an environment favorable to sperm's survival
m. Lubricate urethra and vaginal orifice
n. Division between external and internal female genitals
o. Location for urine to be expelled
p. Narrow, tubular part of the uterus
q. Produces the mucus plug during pregnancy
r. Produces bacteriostatic vaginal lubrication

11. Label the structures of the internal female reproductive organs on the two figures below. Some labels are used more than once. *(23, 24)*

   a. Bartholin's gland
   b. Bladder
   c. Body
   d. Broad ligament
   e. Cervix
   f. Endometrium
   g. Fallopian tube
   h. Fimbriae
   i. Fundus
   j. Infundibulum
   k. Myometrium
   l. Ovary
   m. Perimetrium
   n. Rectum
   o. Rugae
   p. Uterus
   q. Vagina

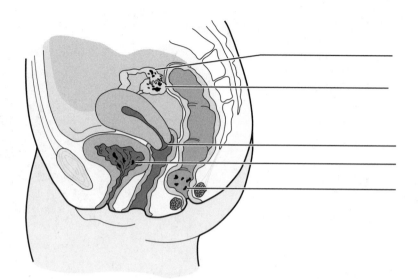

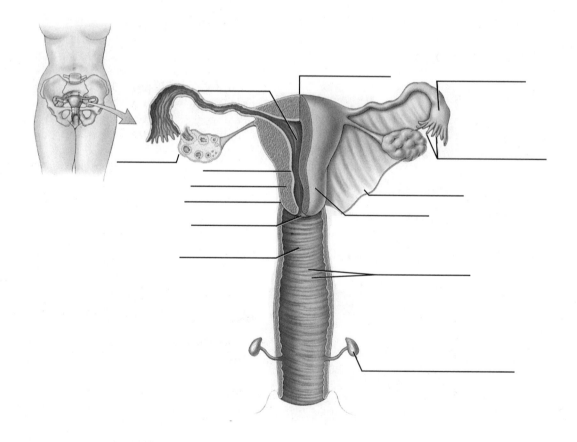

12. Label each diameter of the pelvic inlet on the figure below and list the normal measurements for each. *(26)*

    a. Anteroposterior
    b. Transverse
    c. Left oblique
    d. Right oblique

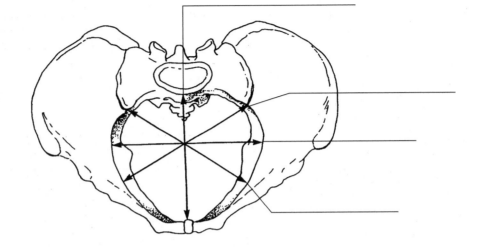

13. Label each structure of the female breast on the figure below. Some labels may be used on both views. *(27)*

    a. Alveolus/alveoli
    b. Areola
    c. Duct
    d. Lactiferous duct
    e. Lactiferous sinus
    f. Nipple
    g. Pectoralis major muscle

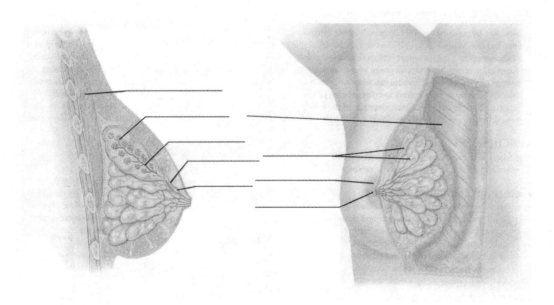

14. Match each female breast structure with its function (a–d). *(27)*

_____	Alveolus/alveoli	a.	Widened area of a duct that holds milk
_____	Areola	b.	Glands that secrete milk
_____	Lactiferous duct	c.	Carry milk from alveoli to nipple
_____	Lactiferous sinus	d.	Area of darker skin surrounding nipple

15. Match each term with its definition (a–e).

_____	Corpus luteum *(27)*	a.	Painful sexual intercourse
_____	Dyspareunia *(23)*	b.	Empty follicle after ovum is released
_____	Follicle *(27)*	c.	First menstrual period
_____	Menarche *(27)*	d.	Release of mature ovum
_____	Ovulation *(27)*	e.	Cavity containing a single ovum

16. State where each of the following female hormones is secreted and its function or functions. *(27)*

a. FSH (follicle-stimulating hormone): _____

   _____

   _____

b. LH (luteinizing hormone): _____

   _____

   _____

c. Estrogen: _____

   _____

   _____

d. Progesterone: _____

   _____

   _____

REVIEW QUESTIONS

1. The average female is usually shorter than the average male because: *(21)*
   1. girls have high levels of testosterone during puberty.
   2. boys begin puberty at an earlier age than girls.
   3. the growth spurt of girls ends earlier than that of boys.
   4. onset of puberty stops growth in a girl's height.

2. A woman can become pregnant even if the male "pulls out" before ejaculation because: *(22)*
   1. ejaculation occurs before insertion of the penis.
   2. some semen is released before ejaculation.
   3. sperm are added to semen after ejaculation.
   4. semen enters the urethra as soon as the penis is inserted.

3. The uterine layer that responds to hormonal changes and receives the fertilized ovum is the: *(24)*
   1. parametrium.
   2. myometrium.
   3. endometrium.
   4. cervicometrium.

4. The true pelvis is divided from the false pelvis by the: *(26)*
   1. obstetric conjugate.
   2. right and left oblique diameters.
   3. linea terminalis.
   4. bi-ischial diameter.

5. Which division of the female pelvis can change slightly to accommodate the fetus during birth? *(25)*
   1. Obstetric conjugate
   2. Right and left oblique diameters
   3. Pelvic outlet
   4. Bischial diameter

6. The function of a male's scrotum is to: *(21)*
   1. regulate the temperature of the testes.
   2. carry sperm from the testes to the penis.
   3. secrete the hormone testosterone.
   4. increase the strength of ejaculation of sperm.

7. The breast structures that secrete milk after childbirth are the: *(27)*
   1. lactiferous ducts.
   2. Montgomery's glands.
   3. alveoli.
   4. nipples.

8. Erection of the penis occurs during sexual stimulation because: *(29)*
   1. smooth muscles attached to the pelvis lift the penis.
   2. blood is trapped within the tissues of the organ.
   3. the testosterone level falls in response to stimulation.
   4. prostate gland secretions cause the organ to stiffen.

9. What is the most appropriate nursing response to the woman who decides she cannot breastfeed because she has small breasts? *(27)*
   1. "Small breasts usually have less milk-secreting tissue, but you could give it a try when the baby arrives."
   2. "Pregnancy hormones will increase most women's breast size enough to feed the average-size infant."
   3. "Small breasts actually have more milk-secreting glands than larger breasts; there should be plenty of milk."
   4. "It is the amount of fat in your breasts that determines their size, so your chances of successfully nursing are good."

10. The middle layer of the myometrium has _____ fibers. *(24)*
    1. circular
    2. figure-eight–shaped
    3. longitudinal
    4. oblique

11. The endometrium of the uterus is thinnest at what time? *(Fig. 2-8, 27)*
    1. Just before ovulation
    2. Between ovulation and menstruation
    3. At the beginning of menstruation
    4. Just after menstruation

THINKING CRITICALLY

1. Your 11-year-old niece confides to you that she is worried because she had her first menstrual period two months ago but has not had another one. She tells you she learned in school that most girls have periods once each month. What would you tell her?

2. A woman is seeing the nurse practitioner because she has recurrent vaginal infections. She says she douches frequently to "keep herself clean," but that the infections often recur, especially when she needs antibiotics, as she is now taking for an ear infection. What advice do you think the nurse would give her? Explain the rationale.

APPLYING KNOWLEDGE

1. Examine a model of the female pelvis. Identify the following landmarks.
   a. Coccyx
   b. Sacrum
   c. Ischial spine
   d. Symphysis pubis
   e. Ilium
   f. Linea terminalis

2. Identify the following pelvic inlet diameters on a model of the female pelvis. Which diameter of the inlet and outlet is the shortest?
   a. Inlet
      i. Anteroposterior
      ii. Left and right oblique
      iii. Transverse
   b. Cavity
      i. Interspinous transverse
   c. Outlet
      i. Anteroposterior
      ii. Intertuberous transverse
      iii. Anteroposterior sagittal

3. Examine a model of the male pelvis. How does the male android pelvis differ from the female gynecoid pelvis?

Fetal Development

Answer Key: A complete answer key can be found on the Student Evolve website.

LEARNING ACTIVITIES

1. Match the terms in the left column with their definitions on the right (a–g).

_____ Diploid *(31)*	a. Normal number of chromosomes in each mature sperm or ovum
_____ Gamete *(32)*	b. Normal number of chromosomes in nonreproductive cells
_____ Haploid *(32)*	
_____ Meiosis *(31)*	c. Cell division in sex cells
_____ Mitosis *(31)*	d. Cell division in non-sex cells to allow growth and replacement of cells
_____ Oogenesis *(31)*	e. Formation of spermatozoa
_____ Spermatogenesis *(31)*	f. Formation of ova
	g. An ovum or spermatozoon

2. a. Spermatogenesis results in the formation of how many sperm from each immature primary sper-matocyte? _____ *(32)*

   b. Each sperm contains _____ autosomes and either a(n) _____ or a(n) _____ sex chromosome. *(31)*

3. a. Oogenesis results in the formation of how many mature ova from each primary oocyte? _____ *(31, 42)*

   b. Each ovum contains _____ autosomes and a(n) _____ sex chromosome. *(31)*

4. a. An ovum survives about _____ hours after ovulation. *(33)*

   b. Sperm survive up to _____ days after ejaculation. *(33)*

5. a. If the ovum is fertilized by a sperm bearing a Y chromosome, the baby will be a _____. *(33-34, Fig. 3-3)*

   b. If the ovum is fertilized by a sperm bearing an X chromosome, the baby will be a _____. *(33-34, Fig. 3-3)*

   c. What influence, if any, does the woman have on the sex of the baby conceived? *(33)* _____

   _____

   _____

6. a. Fertilization usually occurs in the _____ _____. *(33)*

    b. The fertilized ovum usually implants in the _____ section of the _____ uterus. *(33)*

7. Match the terms in the left column with their definitions on the right (a–j).

    _____ Amnion *(35)*

    _____ Blastocyst *(34)*

    _____ Blastomere *(34)*

    _____ Chorion *(35)*

    _____ Decidua basalis *(35)*

    _____ Embryo *(34, 36)*

    _____ Fetus *(36)*

    _____ Morula *(34)*

    _____ Chorionic villi *(35)*

    _____ Zygote *(34, 36)*

    a. Inner fetal membrane that envelops the embryo and fetus
    b. Outer fetal membrane that envelops the amnion and embryo/fetus
    c. Solid cluster of cells that is approximately the same size as the zygote
    d. Eight-cell stage of prenatal development
    e. Projections on the outer part of fetal side of the placenta that extend into the decidua basalis
    f. Prenatal development from the second week until the end of the eighth week after fertilization
    g. Prenatal development from the ninth week after fertilization until birth
    h. Uterine lining after implantation that gives rise to the maternal side of the placenta
    i. Zygote containing an inner cell mass that will develop into the embryo
    j. Cell formed by union of a sperm and ovum

8. The normal amount of amniotic fluid near the end of pregnancy is about _____ mL. *(35)*

9. List the five functions of amniotic fluid. *(35)*

    a. _____

    b. _____

    c. _____

    d. _____

    e. _____

10. Red blood cells are formed by the _____ _____ for the first six weeks after gestation and then are formed by the _____ and _____, and finally the _____ _____. *(35, Table 3-1)*

11. List four functions of the placenta. *(38)*

    a. _____

    b. _____

    c. _____

    d. _____

12. Describe the functions and effects of each of the four placental hormones during pregnancy. *(39)*

    a. Progesterone

    i. _____

    ii. _____

    iii. _____

    iv. _____

    b. Estrogen

    i. _____

    ii. _____

    iii. _____

    iv. _____

    v. _____

    vi. _____

    c. Human chorionic gonadotropin (hCG) _____

    _____

    d. Human placental lactogen (hPL)_____

    _____

13. Label each of the structures listed below on the drawing provided. Color areas to indicate high (red), medium (purple), and low (blue) fetal blood oxygenation. Use the lines on the neonate's illustration on the right to explain how fetal shunts close after birth. *(40; Fig. 3-7)*

    a. Ductus venosus
    b. Ductus arteriosus
    c. Foramen ovale
    d. Umbilical arteries
    e. Umbilical vein

NEONATE

FETUS

14. The umbilical cord should have _____ vein(s) and _____ artery(ies). *(39)*

15. State the age when each fetal circulatory structure closes functionally and permanently. *(40)*

	Functionally	*Permanently*
a. Foramen ovale	_____	_____
b. Ductus arteriosus	_____	_____
c. Ductus venosus	_____	_____

16. Match the prenatal ages with their developmental characteristics on the right (a–h). *(36, Table 3-1)*

_____ 3 weeks	a. Basic structure of all systems established
_____ 6 weeks	b. Possible to monitor fetal status with kick counts
_____ 8 weeks	c. Fetal eyes open
_____ 10 weeks	d. Fetus now considered full-term
_____ 14 weeks	e. Tubular heart begins beating; earliest evidence of brain and spinal cord
_____ 20 weeks	f. External genitalia may be determined by ultrasound
_____ 28 weeks	g. Extremities will move in response to external stimuli
_____ 38 weeks	h. Heart has all four chambers

17. Describe the differences between monozygotic (identical) and dizygotic (fraternal) twins in terms of the following characteristics. *(Fig. 3-8, 41)*

	Characteristic	Monozygotic	Dizygotic
a.	Same sex or different?		
b.	Number of fertilized ova		
c.	Number of placentas		
d.	Number of membranes		
e.	Number of umbilical cords		

REVIEW QUESTIONS

1. Hereditary or genetic traits are passed from one generation to the next within the: *(31)*
   1. chromosomes.
   2. zygote.
   3. chorionic villi.
   4. somatic cells.

2. After six weeks gestation, fetal red blood cells are manufactured in the: *(35, Table 3-1)*
   1. yolk sac.
   2. liver.
   3. bone marrow.
   4. placenta.

3. Which is the outer fetal membrane? *(35)*
   1. Trophoblast
   2. Chorion
   3. Amnion
   4. Yolk sac

4. The primary function of Wharton's jelly is to: *(39)*
   1. keep the three placental blood vessels separated to improve flow.
   2. prevent penetration of a fertilized ovum.
   3. move sperm through the cervix and the uterus and into the fallopian tubes.
   4. carry fetal waste products back to the placenta.

5. Most fetal blood bypasses circulation to the lungs by way of the: *(39)*
   1. ductus venosus.
   2. foramen ovale.
   3. umbilical vein.
   4. umbilical artery.

6. The fetal circulatory structure that carries blood with the lowest oxygen saturation is the: *(39)*
   1. umbilical vein.
   2. umbilical artery.
   3. ductus venosus.
   4. ductus arteriosus.

7. After fertilization, the zygote grows by: *(31)*
   1. meiosis.
   2. mitosis.
   3. oogenesis.
   4. gametogenesis.

8. The primary purpose of amniotic fluid is to: *(35)*
   1. speed maturation of fetal lungs.
   2. prevent cold stress after birth.
   3. protect the fetus during development.
   4. produce hormones to maintain pregnancy.

9. Fetal waste products are disposed of by the: *(38)*
   1. fetal liver.
   2. placenta.
   3. yolk sac.
   4. endoderm.

10. Inadequate progesterone is likely to result in: *(39)*
    1. release of multiple ova.
    2. spontaneous abortion.
    3. persistence of the corpus luteum.
    4. mixture of maternal and fetal blood.

11. Fraternal (dizygotic) twins result when: *(Fig. 3-8, 41)*
    1. they develop from a single fertilized ovum.
    2. two sperm fertilize one ovum.
    3. the embryonic disc does not divide completely.
    4. two sperm fertilize two ova.

12. The sex of identical (monozygotic) twins: *(Fig. 3-8, 41)*
    1. is always the same.
    2. may or may not be the same.
    3. is always different.
    4. is not predictable.

THINKING CRITICALLY

1. A woman comes to the family planning clinic where you work. She wants to try a natural method of birth control rather than use artificial methods of contraception. What facts must you know about the survival time of the ovum and sperm to help your patient effectively use this form of family planning? See also Chapter 2 for information about the menstrual cycle and Chapter 11 for further information about natural family planning.

2. Your friend is disappointed because she has just had her fourth girl. "My husband wants a son so much," she says. "I feel terrible that I can't have a boy for him." What is an appropriate way to respond to your friend? Role play this situation with a classmate to refine your therapeutic communication skills.

APPLYING KNOWLEDGE

1. Examine a placenta, particularly the insertion location of the umbilical cord into the placenta and the cord length.
   a. Identify the following structures.
      i. Amniotic membrane sac (Examine the membrane sacs in a twin placenta if available.)
      ii. Fetal side
      iii. Maternal side
      iv. Umbilical vein
      v. Umbilical arteries (How do the arteries look different from the vein?)
      vi. Wharton's jelly
   b. How does what you see compare with what your text describes as normal? *(38-39)*
   c. Compare what you find in the placenta and cord with what classmates find in the structures they examine.
   d. What variations in the amount of Wharton's jelly did classmates find?

2. Think about multifetal pregnancies and visit the website for the National Center for Health Statistics website: www.cdc.gov/nchs.
   a. What are the changes in the percentage of multifetal deliveries during the past 5 years?
   b. Are any changes associated with infertility therapy?
   c. What is the average age of mothers who have twins or higher-order multiples?

Prenatal Care and Adaptations to Pregnancy

Answer Key: A complete answer key can be found on the Student Evolve website.

LEARNING ACTIVITIES

1. Match the terms in the left column with their definitions on the right (a–g).

   _____ Colostrum *(52)*
   _____ Hemorrhoids *(Table 4-6)*
   _____ Mucous plug *(51)*
   _____ Pseudoanemia *(53)*
   _____ Pica *(61)*
   _____ Spider nevi *(55)*
   _____ Trimester *(48)*

   a. Breast secretion that precedes milk; rich in antibodies
   b. Red elevations of skin with lines radiating from center
   c. Varicose veins of rectum and anus
   d. Anemia occurring because red cells increase less than plasma volume
   e. Ingestion of nonfood substances
   f. 13-week period of pregnancy
   g. Seals cervical canal during pregnancy

2. Match the terms describing a woman's obstetric history with their definitions on the right (a–g). *(47)*

   _____ Abortion
   _____ Gravida
   _____ Multigravida
   _____ Multipara
   _____ Para
   _____ Primigravida
   _____ Primipara

   a. Pregnancy, regardless of duration; pregnant woman
   b. Woman pregnant for the first time
   c. Woman pregnant for the second or subsequent time
   d. Woman who delivered one or more pregnancies after at least 20 weeks gestation
   e. Woman who has delivered one pregnancy of at least 20 weeks gestation
   f. Woman who has delivered two or more pregnancies of at least 20 weeks gestation
   g. End of pregnancy before 20 weeks of gestation

3. Match the signs and symptoms of pregnancy with their descriptions on the right (a–l).

    _____ Abdominal striae *(50; Fig. 4-2)*
    _____ Amenorrhea *(48)*
    _____ Ballottement *(49)*
    _____ Braxton Hicks contractions *(49)*
    _____ Chadwick's sign *(49)*
    _____ Chloasma gravidarum *(49)*
    _____ Funic souffle *(50)*
    _____ Goodell's sign *(49)*
    _____ Hegar's sign *(49)*
    _____ Linea nigra *(49)*
    _____ Quickening *(49)*
    _____ Uterine souffle *(50)*

    a. Bluish color of cervix, vagina, and vulva
    b. Stretch marks
    c. Rebound of fetal part when tapped by examining finger during vaginal examination
    d. Softened lower uterus
    e. Irregular, painless uterine contractions
    f. Blowing sound heard over uterus
    g. Swishing sound of blood circulating through umbilical cord
    h. Cessation of menses
    i. Softened cervix and vagina
    j. Darker-pigmented line in midline of abdomen
    k. Movement of fetus felt by mother
    l. Brownish pigmentation of face ("mask of pregnancy")

4. a. _____ is the hormone detected in a positive pregnancy test. *(48)*

    b. Two body fluids used for pregnancy tests are _____ and _____. *(50)*

5. Describe changes that occur in the reproductive organs during pregnancy. *(51)*

    a. Uterus

        i.   Size:_____
        ii. Weight: _____
        iii. Capacity: _____

    b. Cervix: _____

    c. Ovaries: _____

    d. Vagina:_____

6. Describe changes in other body systems during pregnancy.

    a. Breasts: *(51)*_____

   b. Respiratory: *(52)*_____

_____

_____

   c. Cardiovascular: *(52-53)*_____

_____

_____

   d. Gastrointestinal: *(54)*_____

_____

_____

   e. Urinary: *(54)*_____

_____

_____

   f. Integumentary and skeletal: *(55)*_____

_____

_____

7. Describe the recommended weight gain if the woman's prepregnancy weight is as follows: *(57, 59)*

   a. Normal: _____ to _____ pounds (_____ to _____ kg)

   b. Underweight: _____ to _____ pounds (_____ to _____ kg)

   c. Overweight: _____ to _____ pounds (_____ to _____ kg)

   d. Obese: _____ to _____ pounds (_____ to _____ kg)

8. The recommended calorie increase during pregnancy is _____ kcal per day. During lactation, the recommended calorie increase is _____ kcal per day. *(59)*

9. For the following four nutrients, state the amount needed during pregnancy for an adult and list key food sources for each nutrient. Practice how you would actually teach the information to a pregnant woman. Would you add any information when you teach a breastfeeding woman?

   a. Protein *(60)*

      i. Amount:_____

      ii. Sources: _____

   b. Calcium *(60)*

      i. Amount:_____

      ii. Sources: _____

   c. Iron *(60)*

      i. Amount: _____

      ii. Sources: _____

   d. Folic acid *(61)*

      i. Amount: _____

      ii. Sources: _____

10. Describe how the nurse can help women meet special nutritional needs during pregnancy.

   a. Pregnant adolescent: *(61)* _____

     _____

     _____

   b. Lactose intolerance: *(62)* _____

     _____

     _____

11. List at least three measures the nurse can teach a woman to relieve each common pregnancy discomfort. Note any related abnormal signs or symptoms that should be reported. Practice explaining each relief measure to a pregnant woman. *(65-67; Table 4-6)*

   a. Nausea: _____

     _____

   b. Increased vaginal discharge: _____

     _____

   c. Fatigue: _____

     _____

   d. Backache: _____

     _____

   e. Constipation: _____

     _____

   f. Varicose veins: _____

     _____

   g. Hemorrhoids: _____

     _____

   h. Heartburn: _____

     _____

    i.   Dyspnea and nasal stuffiness: _____

         _____

    j.   Leg cramps:_____

         _____

    k.   Edema of the legs: _____

         _____

12. Describe the common emotional reactions of a woman during each trimester of pregnancy. Describe any of these reactions that you have experienced or witnessed. *(67-68)*

    a.   First: _____

         _____

    b.   Second: _____

         _____

    c.   Third: _____

         _____

REVIEW QUESTIONS

1. A woman who is 20 weeks pregnant is expected to experience: *(67-68)*
   1. nausea and vomiting.
   2. movement of the fetus.
   3. burning during urination.
   4. yellowish vaginal discharge.

2. A woman is 16 weeks pregnant. During a prenatal visit, she tells the nurse she is worried that her baby might not be normal. How should the nurse interpret this statement? *(67-68)*
   1. Concerns about doing "everything right" often become the woman's new standard.
   2. It is unusual for women to have these feelings because they do not perceive the baby as "real."
   3. She may have underlying rejection of the fetus that is being expressed in this way.
   4. Her image of the fetus is not realistic, so the nurse should not be concerned.

3. A woman's emotional reaction during the second trimester of pregnancy may be characterized by: *(68)*
   1. fear for her safety during labor.
   2. passive and dependent behavior.
   3. fantasies about the baby's appearance.
   4. dramatic changes in her moods.

4. While lying on the examining table during her prenatal check at 34 weeks, a woman complains of being dizzy and weak. She is pale and her skin is moist. The best nursing intervention to relieve her symptoms is to: *(53)*
   1. have her turn to her side.
   2. tell her to take deep breaths.
   3. help her sit up on the table.
   4. elevate her feet and legs.

5. To ensure that a woman has adequate iron intake during pregnancy, it is often recommended that she: *(60)*
   1. drink at least one quart of milk per day.
   2. take 30 mg of an iron supplement daily.
   3. eat combinations of meat and grains.
   4. eat 18 mg of iron daily in a variety of foods.

6. What should the nurse teach a pregnant woman about caring for varicose veins in her legs? *(66)*
   1. Apply warm packs to the legs.
   2. Sit down as much as possible.
   3. Stretch the legs while pointing toes.
   4. Elevate the legs when sitting.

7. The primary goal of prenatal care is to assure the woman of: *(44)*
   1. labor with a minimum of pain.
   2. the healthiest outcome possible.
   3. improved long-term nutrition.
   4. minimal pregnancy discomforts.

8. Which foods are the highest in iron? *(60)*
   1. Citrus fruits and melons
   2. Milk, cheese, and other dairy products
   3. Dried beans, potatoes, and legumes
   4. Meat and dark-green vegetables

9. Adequate stores of folic acid are needed before conception to: *(61)*
   1. promote adequate expansion of the blood volume.
   2. reduce nausea and vomiting in the first trimester.
   3. limit depletion of calcium from the mother's teeth.
   4. reduce the risk for fetal neural tube defects.

10. The end outcome (goal) for the nursing diagnosis Altered nutrition: less than body requirements related to low prepregnancy weight, is that the patient will: *(55)*
    1. identify recommended nutrient intake during pregnancy.
    2. gain at least 28 pounds by the end of pregnancy.
    3. recognize that good nutrition promotes maternal and fetal health.
    4. state the appropriate calorie increase for pregnancy.

11. Choose the best intervention to advise a patient to take for relief of constipation during pregnancy. *(65, Table 4-6)*
    1. Take a mild laxative no more than three times per week.
    2. Eat several servings of raw fruits and vegetables each day.
    3. Limit fluids to one quart each day, taken between meals.
    4. Wait until the environment is quiet before defecating.

12. The pregnant woman is more likely to have leg cramps if she: *(66, Table 4-6)*
    1. does not take her iron supplement each day.
    2. increases her fluid intake to eight glasses per day.
    3. stretches each leg while flexing the foot three times each day.
    4. drinks at least 1 to 1.5 quarts of milk each day.

13. A pregnant woman calls the prenatal clinic and says she has a large amount of yellow vaginal discharge. The nurse should instruct the woman to: *(51)*
    1. douche with a commercial vinegar and water solution.
    2. avoid sexual intercourse until the symptoms go away.
    3. wear cotton panties that allow adequate air circulation.
    4. come to the clinic for further evaluation by the midwife.

14. It is important to maintain adequate fluid intake during pregnancy primarily to prevent: *(65, Table 4-6)*
    1. orthostatic hypotension.
    2. edema of the feet and legs.
    3. nausea and vomiting.
    4. urinary tract infection.

CASE STUDIES

1. Rosa comes to the clinic for a regular visit at 26 weeks gestation. Her weight gain has been normal (17 pounds), but she tells you that her mother cautioned her not to gain more than 20 pounds or it will be hard to lose the weight after she gives birth. "My mother said that I should not eat salt and that the doctor will probably give me 'water pills' if I gain too much weight." What teaching should you give Rosa about each of her concerns?
    a. Weight gain
    b. Salt (sodium) intake
    c. Diuretics (water pills)

2. Lauren, 30 years old, is pregnant for the first time. She describes herself as a vegetarian, although she says she occasionally eats dairy products and eggs. What nutritional advice can the nurse provide, considering Lauren's pregnancy needs and her food preferences? *(61, Figure 4-7)*

THINKING CRITICALLY

1. Today is June 19. A woman is admitted to the hospital in labor. She tells you that she has not had prenatal care, but that her "due date" is June 26. How many weeks pregnant is the woman if these dates are confirmed with ultrasound?

2. If a woman's expected date of delivery is July 21, using Nägele's rule in Box 4-2, what was the first day of her last menstrual period?

3. Chelsea, a 15-year-old, arrives at the pregnancy center where you volunteer. She says, "I'm afraid I may be pregnant, but I had sex just one time." You ask her to describe why she thinks she may be pregnant and she lists the symptoms below. State whether each symptom the girl describes is presumptive, probable, or positive. Add nursing actions that assist in knowing which of the three groups describe the girl's symptoms. *(48, Box 4-3)*
    a. Menstrual period is about 10 weeks late.
    b. Breasts are larger than usual and tender when she showers or puts on a bra or tight shirt.
    c. States that she is "getting fat" and feels the need to "pee all the time."
    d. Says that she did a pregnancy test when her period was late, but she is not sure that she "did it right" and wants a repeat test.

APPLYING KNOWLEDGE

1. Have a discussion group that contains both men and women who have had children (they do not have to be nurses or nursing students). Discuss the parts fathers played in any births. Explore the feelings of men in the group about how they view their role in childbirth.

2. Each date below represents the first day of a woman's last menstrual period. Use a wheel to calculate the expected date of delivery for each. If you have access to an electronic gestation calculator, use it to make the same calculations. Using today's date, calculate how many weeks the pregnancy has advanced.
    a. January 18: _____
    b. July 13: _____
    c. December 30: _____

3. Use the TPALM system to describe each of the following pregnancy histories.
    a. A woman is pregnant for the fourth time. She had one spontaneous abortion, one child born at 32 weeks gestation who is living, and another living child born at 41 weeks gestation.
    b. A woman is 32 weeks pregnant with her second pregnancy. Her first pregnancy ended with a spontaneous abortion at 8 weeks gestation.

Nursing Care of Women with Complications During Pregnancy

chapter

5

Answer Key: A complete answer key can be found on the Student Evolve website.

LEARNING ACTIVITIES

1. Match the terms in the left column with their definitions on the right (a–f).

   _____ Abruptio placentae *(88, Table 5-4)*
   _____ Ectopic pregnancy *(86)*
   _____ Hyperemesis gravidarum *(79)*
   _____ Incompetent cervix *(83)*
   _____ Placenta previa *(88, Table 5-4)*
   _____ Spontaneous abortion *(82)*

   a. Placental attachment in the lower uterus
   b. Premature separation of the normally implanted placenta
   c. Spontaneous loss of a pregnancy before 20 weeks (often called *miscarriage*)
   d. Failure of the cervix to remain closed until the fetus is mature enough to survive outside the uterus
   e. Excessive nausea and vomiting during pregnancy
   f. Development of the fetus outside the uterus

2. List at least four appropriate nursing interventions for the woman with hyperemesis gravidarum. *(82)*

   a. _____

   _____

   b. _____

   _____

   c. _____

   _____

   d. _____

   _____

3. Match the types of spontaneous abortion with their descriptions on the right (a–h). *(84; Table 5-2)*

_____ Threatened	a. Bleeding and cramping with cervical dilation but no passage of tissue
_____ Incomplete	b. Bleeding and cramping with passage of some tissue
_____ Inevitable	c. Intentional termination of pregnancy for health reasons
_____ Complete	d. Intentional termination of pregnancy for reasons unrelated to health
_____ Missed	e. Passage of all products of conception
_____ Recurrent	f. Retention of the dead fetus in the uterus
_____ Therapeutic	g. Two or more consecutive spontaneous abortions (also called *habitual abortion*)
_____ Elective	h. Vaginal bleeding without dilation of the cervix or passage of tissue

4. Describe important teaching for a woman after spontaneous abortion for each aspect listed. *(85)*

    a. Bleeding: _____

    _____

    b. Temperature: _____

    _____

    c. Iron supplementation: _____

    _____

    d. Resuming sexual activity: _____

    _____

    e. Contraception: _____

    _____

5. An ectopic pregnancy usually occurs in the _____ _____. *(86)*

6. The priority nursing observation related to ectopic pregnancy is for _____ _____. *(87)*

7. Describe each characteristic of gestational trophoblastic disease, also called *hydatidiform mole* or *molar pregnancy*. *(87)*

    a. Bleeding: _____

    _____

    b. Uterine size: _____

    _____

   c.   Fetal heart activity: _____

       _____

   d.   Presence of vomiting: _____

       _____

   e.   Blood pressure:_____

       _____

   f.   Human chorionic gonadotropin (hCG) levels: _____

       _____

   g.   Ultrasound appearance: _____

       _____

   h.   Risk for cancer:_____

       _____

8.   Describe the location of each type of placenta previa. *(88; Table 5-4)*

   a.   Marginal:_____

       _____

   b.   Partial: _____

       _____

   c.   Total: _____

       _____

9. How does placenta previa compare to abruptio placentae in each of the following characteristics? *(88; Table 5-4)*

	Placenta Previa	Abruptio Placentae
a. Pain		
b. Characteristics of bleeding		
c. Fetal anemia and/or hypoxia		
d. Consistency of the uterus		
e. Blood coagulation		
f. Risk for postpartum hemorrhage		
g. Risk for postpartum infection		

10. Using the Patient Teaching box on p. 92, list the factors that suggest development of gestational hypertension (GH) and the possible cause of each. Put an X next to those that suggest a seizure may occur soon if there is no intervention. *(90-91)*

_____

_____

_____

_____

_____

_____

_____

_____

11. List six or more factors that increase a woman's risk for development of GH. *(91; Box 5-3)*

    a. _____

    b. _____

    c. _____

    d. _____

    e. _____

    f. _____

12. Describe each variation of hypertensive disorders of pregnancy. *(90; Table 5-5)*

    a. Gestational hypertension:_____

    _____

    b. Preeclampsia: _____

    _____

    c. Eclampsia:_____

    _____

    d. HELLP: _____

    _____

    e. Chronic hypertension:_____

    _____

    f. Preeclampsia with superimposed chronic hypertension: _____

    _____

13. What blood pressure elevation is significant during pregnancy? *(90; Table 5-5)* _____

_____

14. Describe manifestations of preeclampsia and the cause of each. Note those that suggest severe preeclampsia. *(90-92)*

   a. Hypertension:_____

   _____

   b. Edema:_____

   _____

   c. Proteinuria: _____

   _____

   d. Central nervous system changes: _____

   _____

   e. Visual disturbances:_____

   _____

   f. Urine output: _____

   _____

   g. Pulmonary edema: _____

   _____

   h. Epigastric pain (upper abdominal, over stomach) or nausea: _____

   _____

   i. Lab study abnormalities (liver enzymes, coagulation):_____

   _____

15. What is the benefit of activity restriction in treatment of preeclampsia? *(92)* _____

   _____

16. a. What is the purpose of magnesium sulfate in the treatment of hypertension? *(92)* _____

   _____

   b. What observations are needed for a woman who is receiving magnesium sulfate as treatment for hypertension? *(92-93)*

   _____

   c. What drug should be on hand if a woman is receiving magnesium sulfate? *(93)*_____

   _____

   d. What is the desired serum level of magnesium when treating a woman with hypertension? *(93)*

   _____

17. a. Rh blood incompatibility can only occur if the mother is Rh _____ and the fetus is Rh
      _____. *(95)*

    b. The drug given to prevent Rh incompatibility is _____. *(95)*

    c. List four instances in which the drug listed in part (b) is indicated. *(95)*

       i. _____

       ii. _____

       iii. _____

       iv. _____

18. Which type of diabetes occurs only during pregnancy? *(96, 97)* _____

19. Describe the test used to screen for gestational diabetes and the normal results. When is screening done?
    (97)

    _____

    _____

20. a. Why is glucose monitored more frequently by blood testing during pregnancy than when a woman
      is not pregnant? *(98-99; Nursing Care Plan 5-3)*

      _____

      _____

    b. What place does urine testing have in diabetes management during pregnancy? *(Table 5-7; Nursing
      Care Plan 5-3)*

      _____

      _____

21. The preferred drug used to control the blood glucose during pregnancy is _____
    because it _____. *(100)*

22. Describe how insulin requirements change during the course of pregnancy and after birth. *(100)*

    _____

    _____

23. How may exercise needs differ in the woman who has preexisting diabetes and the woman with gesta-
    tional diabetes? *(100)*

    _____

    _____

24. How may the normal changes of pregnancy affect the woman with heart disease? *(101)* _____

    _____

    _____

25. How do labor and the postpartum period change the demands on the heart? *(101)*_____

_____

_____

26. List three reasons why a pregnant woman needs increased iron. *(102)*

    a. _____

    b. _____

    c. _____

27. A woman who is 25 weeks pregnant with her first child has her first prenatal visit. Her initial hemoglobin is 10.8 g/dL. What is the appropriate nursing response to this lab value? *(102-103)*

_____

_____

_____

28. List foods high in the following nutrients. *(Nutrition Considerations, p. 103)*

    a. Iron: _____

    _____

    b. Folic acid: _____

    _____

    c. Vitamin C:_____

    _____

29. a. What types of foods are good to take with an iron supplement and why? *(103)* _____

    _____

    b. What foods or drugs should be avoided at the time an iron supplement is taken and why? *(103)*

    _____

    _____

30. What are the differences in supplementation of folic acid for routine prevention and actual folic acid deficiency? *(102)*

_____

_____

_____

31. What is the effect of a sickle cell crisis during pregnancy? *(102-103)* _____

_____

32. Match each maternal infection with the method to prevent infection of the fetus or newborn on the right (a–f).

_____ Cytomegalovirus *(103)*

_____ Rubella *(103)*

_____ Herpes virus *(103)*

_____ Hepatitis B *(103)*

_____ Toxoplasmosis *(106)*

_____ Group B streptococcus *(106)*

a. Deliver infant by cesarean birth if the woman has genital lesions when labor begins

b. Give immune globulin immediately after birth followed by vaccine

c. Immunize children to avoid infecting pregnant women; immunize nonimmune woman after birth

d. Treat culture-positive woman and her infant with penicillin

e. Wash hands and surfaces after handling raw meat, cook meat thoroughly, avoid cat litter

f. No effective prevention or treatment

33. What are the recommendations to prevent hepatitis B in the newborn? *(104)* _____

_____

_____

34. List three ways an infant may be infected with human immunodeficiency virus (HIV). *(105; Box 5-7)*

a. _____

b. _____

c. _____

35. What teaching about the following is appropriate to reduce the spread of HIV? *(105)*

a. Drug abuse:_____

b. Vaginal intercourse:_____

c. Oral sex:_____

36. Why is a pregnant woman more likely to have a urinary tract infection? *(107)* _____

_____

_____

37. List at least three things the nurse can teach a woman about avoiding a urinary tract infection. *(107)*

a. _____

b. _____

c. _____

38. Describe general approaches to the care of pregnant women related to bioterrorist attacks. *(107-108)*

_____

_____

_____

39. a.   Describe the manifestations of fetal alcohol syndrome (FAS). *(108; Fig. 5-8)* _____

    _____

    _____

   b.   What is the current recommendation about alcohol intake during pregnancy? *(109; Table 5-9)*

    _____

    _____

40. Match each substance with its potential adverse effects when used during pregnancy or appropriate preventive measures (a–i). *(109; Table 5-9)*

_____ ACE inhibitors	a. Abstinence syndrome may develop in woman or infant if drug is stopped suddenly
_____ Cigarette smoking	b. Associated with congenital heart disease and toxicity to fetal thyroid and kidneys
_____ Cocaine	c. Causes spontaneous abortion and other serious fetal anomalies
_____ Folic acid antagonists	d. Crosses placenta, possibly causing spontaneous abortion, growth restriction, and central nervous system and facial defects
_____ Heroin	
_____ Lithium	e. Fetal kidney abnormalities, growth restriction, and insufficient amniotic fluid
_____ Tetracycline	f. Infant may be smaller than expected for gestation
_____ Vitamin A preparations (isotretinoin [Accutane])	g. Infant may have discolored teeth
_____ Warfarin	h. Reliable birth control is needed for 3 months after treatment with this drug
	i. Severe vasoconstriction may cause preterm labor, hypertension with reduced placental circulation, and maternal stroke

41. If a woman needs a potentially teratogenic therapeutic drug during pregnancy, how will her health care provider make a decision about what to prescribe? *(110)*

    _____

    _____

42. What are three potential risks to a woman and her infant if she is a victim of physical abuse? *(110)*

   a.   _____

   b.   _____

   c.   _____

43. List common manifestations of battering. *(111)* _____

    _____

    _____

    _____

REVIEW QUESTIONS

1. A pregnant woman with type 1 diabetes mellitus asks the nurse why she has needed several increases in her insulin dose during pregnancy. The best answer is that the: *(96-97)*
    1. pregnancy changes decrease the secretion of insulin from the pancreas.
    2. placenta secretes substances that reduce the effectiveness of insulin.
    3. fetus does not yet secrete insulin and needs more from the mother.
    4. pancreas secretes progressively less insulin as pregnancy progresses.

2. The purpose of the biophysical profile (BPP) is to: *(81; Table 5-1)*
    1. assess any Rh blood incompatibility between the mother and fetus.
    2. determine if the fetal lungs are mature enough to survive extrauterine life.
    3. determine if the placenta is functioning well enough to support fetal life.
    4. identify serious congenital abnormalities during early pregnancy.

3. If a pregnant woman is not immune to rubella, the expected action is to: *(104)*
    1. limit her contact with other pregnant women.
    2. immunize her early in the postpartum period.
    3. inform her that her baby may have defects.
    4. tell her that there is little risk for problems.

4. Select the most appropriate teaching for the woman who is prone to urinary tract infections. *(107)*
    1. Wipe the perineal area in a front-to-back direction.
    2. Eat a diet high in fiber, iron, and vitamin C.
    3. Eat a diet that includes additional citrus fruits and drinks.
    4. Avoid using added lubricant during sexual intercourse.

5. If a woman has cardiac disease, the main risks to the fetus are related to: *(101; Box 5-5)*
    1. poor oxygenation.
    2. preterm birth.
    3. maternal infection.
    4. congenital anomalies.

6. Which fetal or neonatal problem should the nurse anticipate if a woman has persistent hyperemesis gravidarum? *(79)*
    1. Multiple vitamin and mineral deficiencies
    2. Poor attachment behaviors at birth
    3. Smaller than expected birth weight
    4. Neonatal sepsis

7. Choose the maternal sign or symptom that is most characteristic of hypovolemic shock associated with blood loss in a pregnant woman. *(86; Box 5-1)*
    1. Oral temperature below 36.1° C (97° F)
    2. Abnormal uterine contractions
    3. Urine output of 100 mL/hour
    4. Weak pulse that increases in rate

8. Choose the assessment that should be promptly reported to the physician when a woman is being observed in the emergency department for possible ectopic pregnancy. *(86; Box 5-1)*
    1. Hypertension with deep, irregular respirations
    2. Light vaginal bleeding without cramping
    3. Bradycardia with cyanosis
    4. Fall in urine output to 20 mL/hour

9. The nurse should emphasize the importance of long-term follow-up care for the woman who has had evacuation of a hydatidiform mole to detect the occurrence of: *(87)*
   1. recurrent pregnancy.
   2. choriocarcinoma.
   3. hypertension.
   4. continued bleeding.

10. A significant difference between the signs of abruptio placentae and those of placenta previa is that abruptio placentae involves: *(88; Table 5-4)*
    1. dark or concealed bleeding.
    2. some uterine irritation.
    3. infection.
    4. vomiting.

11. A woman who has been monitored for vaginal bleeding related to suspected placenta previa has a viable fetus that may have fetal anemia as a result. Which test should the nurse expect? *(88; Table 5-4)*
    1. X-ray
    2. Vaginal exam
    3. Alpha-fetoprotein
    4. Percutaneous umbilical blood sampling

12. A woman who is hospitalized with severe preeclampsia should be closely observed for the onset of: *(90, 92)*
    1. seizures.
    2. decreased uric acid levels.
    3. hypotension.
    4. polyuria.

13. Patient education for the woman who has active herpes virus infection during pregnancy should include: *(104)*
    1. antibiotic treatment of the baby after birth.
    2. the possibility of birth by cesarean delivery.
    3. minor local effects of herpes infection on a newborn.
    4. that immunity is permanent after initial infection.

14. The nurse should expect to teach the pregnant woman with gestational diabetes to monitor her glucose by: *(100; Table 5-7)*
    1. assessing blood levels several times a day.
    2. determining levels in the urine twice a day.
    3. recording monthly glycosylated hemoglobin levels.
    4. keeping a written record of hypoglycemic symptoms.

15. Teaching for the pregnant woman who was newly diagnosed with tuberculosis should include: *(106-107)*
    1. increasing fluid intake to 2 quarts each day.
    2. the expectation that birth will require a cesarean delivery.
    3. the importance of taking the entire course of medication.
    4. remain hospitalized and avoid contact with family members until all medication is taken.

16. To improve circulation to the placenta in a pregnant woman who has been in a serious car accident, the nurse should: *(111)*
    1. place the woman in a slight head-down position on a horizontal surface.
    2. give all intravenous fluids by pump to reduce fluid overload on her heart.
    3. take vital signs every 15 minutes if her condition is not stable.
    4. place a small pillow under one hip if she must lie on her back.

CASE STUDY

1. Amy, a 28-year-old, is pregnant for the fifth time. She has had two spontaneous abortions and one still-born baby who was born at 35 weeks gestation. Amy's only living child, Sam, weighed 10 pounds, 3 ounces when born at 36 weeks gestation. Amy had hypertension in her pregnancy with Sam and with her stillborn baby. She is at the clinic for her first prenatal visit at about 20 weeks. An ultrasound accurately determines the gestational age to be 25 weeks. The nurse practitioner determines that Amy began pregnancy about 25 pounds overweight, although her weight gain is normal for 25 weeks. Initial prenatal checks are normal.
   a. Identify three or more factors that predispose Amy to complications in this pregnancy. Can any of the risk factors be modified safely? What prenatal assessments may identify these complications early? What danger signals in pregnancy should you teach Amy?
   b. Amy's pregnancy progresses normally until 28 weeks gestation. Both the glucose screen (glucose challenge test) and a glucose tolerance test were abnormal, and Amy must take insulin injections twice a day to control her gestational diabetes. What teaching will Amy need for this new problem?
   c. Is there a possibility that her diabetes may not be limited to gestational? Why? When is the health care provider likely to know that Amy's diabetes is a different type?
   d. Amy is now 35 weeks pregnant. Her gestational diabetes has been well-controlled, although she has needed higher doses of insulin as pregnancy progressed. She has now developed mild preeclampsia, and her health care provider admits her to the high-risk pregnancy unit to identify the best therapy for her and the baby. What basic teaching and care are appropriate? How can the nursing staff help Amy and her family cope with the stresses of high-risk pregnancy? What role would an LPN/LVN have in high-risk pregnancy care in your clinical facility?

THINKING CRITICALLY

1. How might anemia affect a woman who has heart disease?

2. You are helping to care for a woman receiving intravenous magnesium sulfate. You note that her urine output has decreased, and was 20 mL during the past hour. What is the significance of your observation? What is the appropriate action? Why?

3. If a couple loses a baby at 8 weeks because of spontaneous abortion (miscarriage), how do you think their friends and family are likely to react? What emotional support is appropriate if the woman believes that she should not feel sad because she did not really know the baby yet? How can the nurse help the family cope with this crisis? (These questions can also be enacted by a small group and show both therapeutic and nontherapeutic responses by the nurse. Some group members may be willing to relate personal experiences with a pregnancy loss.)

APPLYING KNOWLEDGE

1. Assist the experienced nurse in assessing each of these reflexes. Will any of these be inaccurate when a woman has epidural analgesia or anesthesia for birth?
   a. Patellar
   b. Biceps
   c. Triceps
   d. Radial

2. Study your hospital's policies and procedures for nursing care related to magnesium sulfate therapy for preeclampsia or eclampsia.

3. Observe the nursing care of a woman who is receiving magnesium sulfate for GH. What is the reason for each nursing intervention specifically related to magnesium sulfate administration? Did the woman have any of the risk factors for GH listed in Box 5-3 in the textbook?

4. What foods in your usual diet provide adequate folic acid?

Nursing Care of Mother and Infant During Labor and Birth

Answer Key: A complete answer key can be found on the Student Evolve website.

LEARNING ACTIVITIES

1. List the "4 Ps" of the birth process. *(119)*

   a. _____

   b. _____

   c. _____

   d. _____

2. The two powers of labor are _____ _____ and _____
   _____. *(119)*

3. a. Cervical effacement is expressed as _____
   _____. *(120; Fig 6-2)*

   b. The amount of cervical dilation is expressed in _____. *(120; Fig 6-3)*

4. a. The nurse should promptly report contraction durations longer than _____ seconds or intervals shorter than _____ seconds and a frequency closer than every _____ minutes.

   b. Why? *(120, Box 6-3)* _____
   _____
   _____

5. State two reasons why the sutures and fontanelles of the fetal head are important in the birth process. *(122)*

   a. _____
   _____

   b. _____
   _____

6. The abbreviations below describe fetal presentation and position. Spell out each and identify the one describing a breech presentation, the one describing a face presentation, and the one that is the most common of those listed. Identify the fetal presentation and position that often cause "back labor" during birth. *(124-125; Box 6-1; Figure 6-8)*

   a. RSA: _____

   b. LMT: _____

   c. ROA: _____

   d. LOP: _____

7. The key difference between true labor and false labor is _____
   _____. *(131; Table 6-2)*

8. List the three phases of the first stage of labor. Describe cervical changes and the approximate duration of each phase. *(144; Table 6-6)*

   a. _____

   _____

   b. _____

   _____

   c. _____

   _____

9. Describe typical maternal behaviors or occurrences during each stage and phase of labor. Describe any behavioral changes you noted during clinical when caring for a laboring woman. Was an epidural administered at any point? What behavioral changes did you note with that intervention? *(144-145; Table 6-6)*

   a. First stage

      i. Latent phase: _____

      _____

      ii. Active phase: _____

      _____

      iii. Transition phase: _____

      _____

   b. Second stage: _____

   _____

   c. Third stage: _____

   _____

   d. Fourth stage: _____

   _____

10. Describe characteristics of the normal fetal heart rate at term. *(132; Skill 6-2; 135; Box 6-3)*

    Rate: _____ (lower limit) to _____ (upper limit)

    Other characteristics: _____

    _____

11. Describe three characteristics of abnormal amniotic fluid. *(137)*_____

    _____

    _____

12. Describe the assessments in the following categories that the nurse should promptly report when caring for a laboring woman. *(132, 135; Skill 6-2; Box 6-3)*

    a. Temperature:_____

    b. Blood pressure:_____

    c. Fetal heart rate:_____

REVIEW QUESTIONS

1. A baseline fetal heart rate of 125 bpm during labor should be interpreted as: *(132; Skill 6-2)*
   1. normal for a term fetus.
   2. abnormal if the fetus is preterm.
   3. high normal when in labor.
   4. a slow baseline fetal heart rate.

2. When assessing the duration of labor contractions by palpation, the nurse should time from the: *(135; Skill 6-5)*
   1. beginning of one contraction to the end of the same contraction.
   2. end of one contraction to the beginning of the next.
   3. beginning of one contraction to the beginning of the next.
   4. peak of one contraction to the end of the contraction.

3. During normal labor, contractions characteristically become: *(120-121; 128; 131, Table 6-2; 139, Skill 6-5)*
   1. more frequent and of shorter duration.
   2. more frequent and of longer duration.
   3. less frequent and of shorter duration.
   4. less frequent and of longer duration.

4. When the fetus is in a cephalic presentation, the amniotic fluid is expected to be: *(137)*
   1. cloudy.
   2. clear.
   3. green.
   4. yellow.

5. The thinning of the cervix during labor is called: *(120)*
   1. dilation.
   2. effacement.
   3. station.
   4. presentation.

6. How should the nurse interpret the abbreviation *ROP*? *(124-125, Fig. 6-8)*
   1. The fetal sacrum is in the mother's right posterior pelvis.
   2. The fetal pelvis is in the mother's right occipital pelvis.
   3. The fetal occiput is in the mother's right posterior pelvis.
   4. The right fetal occiput is in the mother's posterior pelvis.

7. The labor phase when the woman often feels anxious, restless, and seems to lose control is: *(144, Table 6-6)*
   1. latent.
   2. active.
   3. transition.
   4. placental.

8. Thirty minutes after birth, the nurse assesses the woman's uterine fundus. It is firm, above her umbilicus, and deviated to the right side. The appropriate nursing action is to: *(144, Table 6-6)*
   1. massage the uterus.
   2. assist her to urinate.
   3. provide mild analgesia.
   4. restrict oral intake.

9. Choose the abbreviation that describes the fetus in a breech presentation. *(124-125; 133, Fig. 6-12)*
   1. LSA
   2. LOA
   3. ROA
   4. FHR

10. Which sign or symptom normally occurs shortly before labor begins? *(126)*
    1. An urge to push or bear down
    2. Increased clear vaginal discharge
    3. Moderate amount of vaginal bleeding
    4. Sudden weight gain of 3–5 pounds

11. Fetal descent during labor is measured in relation to the mother's: *(126)*
    1. posterior perineum.
    2. sacral promontory.
    3. ischial spines.
    4. uterine fundus.

12. When the placenta is delivered with the fetal side presenting, the mechanism is called: *(145, 147, Fig. 6-22)*
    1. Duncan.
    2. Lamaze.
    3. VBAC.
    4. Schultze.

13. During the latent phase of labor, the nurse should expect the woman's behavior to be: *(144, Table 6-6)*
    1. sleepy, except during contractions.
    2. mildly anxious, coping with contractions.
    3. quiet, concentrating on each contraction.
    4. frustrated, losing control with contractions.

14. A woman's membranes rupture during labor. The nurse notes that the fluid is yellowish and cloudy. The priority nursing response related to this assessment is to: *(137)*
    1. remove wet underpads and replace them with dry ones.
    2. perform a vaginal examination to assess labor progress.
    3. reassure the woman that membrane rupture is expected.
    4. assess the woman's temperature and the fetal heart rate.

15. The nurse should learn to evaluate labor progress by methods other than vaginal examination, primarily because vaginal examination: *(138)*
    1. worsens the mother's discomfort.
    2. increases the risk for infection.
    3. reduces fetal heart rate variability.
    4. delays normal progression of labor.

16. Of the following, which is the priority for nursing care during the second stage of labor? *(143, Safety Alert; 144, Table 6-6)*
    1. Observe the woman's perineum.
    2. Encourage pushing with contractions.
    3. Evaluate labor coping skills.
    4. Administer ordered analgesia.

17. Which maternal position should be avoided during labor? *(136, 137)*
    1. Sitting
    2. Walking
    3. Side-lying
    4. Supine

18. The woman having a vaginal birth after cesarean (VBAC) should be observed during labor, particularly for signs of: *(143)*
    1. labor progression.
    2. uterine rupture.
    3. perineal pressure.
    4. excessive anxiety.

19. Which nursing assessment finding should be promptly reported to the physician or nurse-midwife? *(135, Box 6-3; 139, Skill 6-5)*
    1. Clear amniotic fluid containing white flecks
    2. Fetal heart rate of 145 bpm with variability
    3. Vaginal discharge of mucus with dark blood
    4. Contraction intervals shorter than 2 minutes

20. The priority nursing observation during the fourth stage of labor is for: *(144, Table 6-6)*
    1. vaginal bleeding.
    2. perineal bulging.
    3. uterine infection.
    4. parent-infant bonding.

21. When assessing labor contractions, the nurse notes that the contracting uterus can be slightly indented with the fingertips when contractions are at their peak. Contraction intensity should be recorded as: *(139, Skill 6-5)*
    1. mild.
    2. moderate.
    3. firm.
    4. latent.

22. A woman phones the birth center and says, "I think my water broke and my baby is due, but I'm not having any contractions." The most appropriate nursing response is to tell her that: *(126)*
    1. labor should begin within a few hours at most.
    2. urine leakage may be confused with ruptured membranes.
    3. she should come to the birth center for evaluation.
    4. there is no concern unless the fluid is bloody.

23. Amniotic fluid usually turns a pH swab or paper: *(137)*
    1. yellow.
    2. green.
    3. dark blue.
    4. purple.

24. The nurse notes a pattern of variable decelerations on the electronic fetal monitor strip. The initial nursing response should be to: *(137)*
    1. reassure the woman that the pattern is expected.
    2. change the laboring woman's position.
    3. increase the rate of the nonadditive IV fluid.
    4. notify the physician of the abnormal pattern.

25. The primary means of identifying hemorrhage after vaginal birth is to: *(147)*
    1. assess vital signs frequently.
    2. observe the uterine fundus and lochia.
    3. keep an ice pack on the perineum.
    4. have the woman urinate every 2 hours.

26. The term infant may be placed in skin-to-skin contact with the mother immediately after birth primarily for the purpose of: *(129, Skill 6-1; also see 150)*
    1. breastfeeding while the baby is alert.
    2. maintaining the infant's temperature.
    3. promoting early parent-infant attachment.
    4. stimulating expulsion of the placenta.

CROSSWORD PUZZLE

Across
2. Bending of the fetal head toward the chest during labor *(124, Fig. 6-7)*
4. Downward progression of the fetal presenting part *(126)*
6. Fetal flexion or extension *(122)*
9. Strength of labor contractions *(144, Table 6-6)*
10. Part of the true pelvis that is nearest the perineum *(122)*
12. Time from the beginning of one contraction until the beginning of the next *(139, Skill 6-5)*
13. Upper part of the true pelvis *(122)*
15. Fetal part that enters pelvis first *(122)*
16. Orientation of the fetus in relation to the mother's spine *(122)*
18. Level of the fetal presenting part in relation to the ischial spines in the pelvis *(126)*
20. Thinning of the cervix *(120)*

22. Fetal substance that may normally be found in amniotic fluid *(137)*
23. Opening of the cervix *(120)*
25. Orientation of a fixed point on the fetus to the mother's pelvis *(123)*
27. Descent of the fetal presenting part to a zero station or lower *(126)*
30. Relaxation period between two labor contractions *(121)*

Down
1. Stage of labor from the baby's birth until delivery of the placenta *(145, Table 6-6)*
2. Stage of labor from its onset to complete cervical dilation *(145, Table 6-6)*
3. Birth of the fetal shoulders and body *(128)*
4. Length of a labor contraction from its beginning to its end *(120)*
5. Characteristic of normal amniotic fluid *(137)*

7. Amniotic fluid may be cloudy if this condition is present *(137)*
8. Period of decreasing strength of a labor contraction *(120)*
9. Fetal rotation as the head turns within the mother's pelvis *(126)*
11. Lower portion of pelvis *(122)*
14. Fontanelle that has three suture lines leading into it *(122; 123, Fig. 6-5)*
17. Fetal rotation as the head turns to face one of the mother's thighs *(128)*
19. Period of increasing strength of a labor contraction *(120)*

21. Middle part of the true pelvis *(122)*
24. Pivoting of fetal head under the mother's symphysis pubis during labor *(127)*
25. Period of greatest strength of a labor contraction *(139, Skill 6-5)*
26. Maternal pushing occurs during this stage of labor *(145, Table 6-6)*
28. Fontanelle that has four suture lines leading to it *(122; 123, Fig. 6-5)*
29. Upper flaring part of the mother's pelvis *(122)*

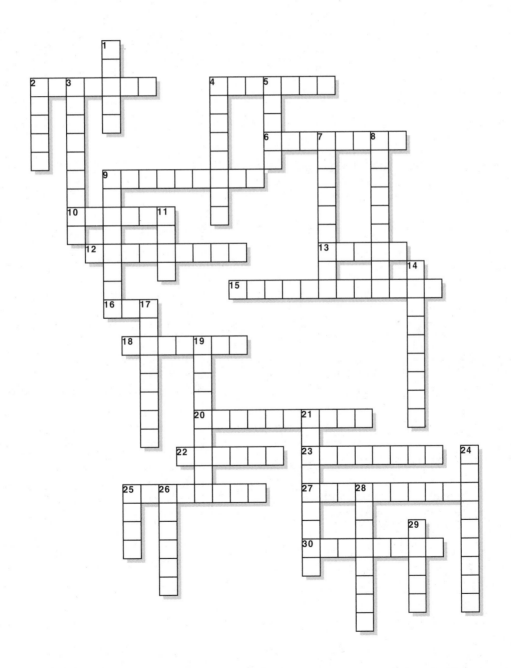

CASE STUDIES

1. A nurse working in a prenatal clinic must teach a woman who does not speak the same language when to go to the hospital. The woman is having her third baby, the first in the United States. Her first labor lasted 18 hours and her second labor lasted 6 hours. What should the nurse teach this woman? Give a rationale for each part of your teaching.

2. A woman is in labor with her first baby. Her cervix is dilated 7 cm, and the fetal station is +1. Formulate appropriate nursing interventions for the nursing diagnosis Acute pain related to labor process and exertion of labor.

THINKING CRITICALLY

1. The following chart shows a typical status report often used in intrapartum units. Interpret the data about each woman's labor by answering the questions below.

Name	Gravida	Para	Gest	Dil	Eff	Sta	FHR
Amy	2	0	36	1–2	50%	–2	160
Becky	4	3	42	6	80%	–1	115
Cathy	1	0	40	3–4	90%	0	144
Deanna	3	1	39	C	C	+2	132

   a. Which patient(s) is/are at full-term gestation?
   b. Which fetus(es) is/are engaged?
   c. Who is likely to deliver soonest? Why?

2. Calculate the 1- and 5-minute Apgar scores on the following infants. *(152, Table 6-7)*

Sign	Baby boy		Twin A (girl)		Twin B (girl)	
	1 min	*5 min*	*1 min*	*5 min*	*1 min*	*5 min*
Heart rate	125	155	88	130	110	90
Respiratory effort	Strong cry	Reacts spontaneously	Weak cry	Strong cry	Weak cry	Weak cry
Muscle tone	Flexed body	Maintains flexion	Limp	Sluggish movement	Sluggish movement	Sluggish movement
Reflex irritability	Cries and flexes body when suctioned	Cries when suctioned or stimulated	Minimal response to suction	Cries when suctioned or stimulated	Active movement when suctioned	Minimal response to suction
Color	Pink body, blue hands and feet	Pink body, blue hands and feet	Pale	Pink body, blue hands and feet	Pink body, blue hands and feet	Blue body and extremities
Total Scores	a.	b.	c.	d.	e.	f.

3. What is the primary reason for closely observing the maternal bladder immediately after birth? *(145, Table 6-6; 147)*

4. What is the significance of the following patterns on the electronic fetal monitor? Include the nursing response to each, as appropriate. *(132; Skill 6-2; Box 6-3)*
    a. Variability
    b. Accelerations
    c. Early decelerations
    d. Variable decelerations
    e. Late decelerations

APPLYING KNOWLEDGE

1. Use a model of a pelvis and fetal head to place the head in each of the following positions. Move the head through each mechanism of labor for each of the positions.

a. ROA	d. LOA	f. LOP
b. ROT	e. LOT	g. OA
c. ROP		

2. During your clinical experience, note how different fetal presentations or positions affect the woman's comfort during labor. Note if there is an apparent effect on the length of labor.

3. Palpate the uterine contractions of women in labor and classify them as mild, moderate, or firm intensity. Confirm your observations with an experienced intrapartum nurse.

4. Observe the labor of a woman having a vaginal birth after cesarean (VBAC) for the following factors related to her experience.
    a. Number of previous cesarean and vaginal births
    b. Reason for previous cesarean birth
    c. The woman's desire to have this baby vaginally
    d. Maternal behaviors during labor
    e. Support of her partner
    f. Her apparent feelings after birth, whether it was VBAC or a repeat cesarean

5. Examine electronic fetal monitor strips to identify the following features:
    a. Information that the monitor automatically prints on the strip or the screen
    b. Interface with computer device, if any
    c. Differences in appearance between results obtained with external devices and those from internal devices
    d. Presence or absence of variability, rate accelerations, and deceleration patterns
    e. Nursing and medical responses to abnormal patterns; fetal response to interventions
    f. Outcome of birth, including Apgar scores of the infant

6. Locate the "precip tray" (which may have a different name) in your clinical facility. What are the contents of this tray?

Nursing Management of Pain During Labor and Birth

Answer Key: A complete answer key can be found on the Student Evolve website.

LEARNING ACTIVITIES

1. Match the terms in the left column with their definitions on the right (a–e).

   _____ Effleurage *(162; Fig 7-2; Box 7-1)*
   _____ Endorphins *(160)*
   _____ Focal point *(162; Box 7-1)*
   _____ Pain threshold *(159)*
   _____ Pain tolerance *(159)*

   a. Least amount of stimulation that a person perceives as painful
   b. Maximum amount of pain one is willing to bear
   c. Stroking of the abdomen, thighs, or other body parts
   d. Intense concentration on an object
   e. Internal substances similar to morphine

2. List four physical factors that cause pain during labor. *(159)*

   a. _____

   b. _____

   c. _____

   d. _____

3. How do each of these physical factors influence a woman's pain during labor? *(159-161)*

   a. Cervical readiness:_____

   _____

   b. Pelvic size and shape: _____

   _____

   c. Labor intensity: _____

   _____

   d. Maternal fatigue: _____

   _____

   e. Fetal presentation and position: _____

   _____

4. How does a woman's anxiety or fear relate to labor pain? *(161)*_____

_____

_____

5. How can each aspect of prenatal classes help a woman in labor? *(158-159; Box 7-1)*

   a. Education about expected changes: _____

   _____

   b. Conditioning exercise:_____

   _____

   c. Identify classes offered at your clinical facility, who teaches them, and the classes that continue after birth.

   _____

   _____

6. List three reasons why it is useful for any laboring woman to know nonpharmacologic pain control methods. *(161)*

   a. _____

   b. _____

   c. _____

7. a. Explain why promoting a woman's relaxation during labor is essential to any type of pain management. *(162)*

   _____

   _____

   b. Describe at least four ways to help the laboring woman relax. *(162-163)*_____

   _____

   _____

   _____

   _____

8. What nursing care may help a woman cope with the following problems during labor?

   a. Hyperventilation: *(164; Box 7-2)* _____

   _____

   b. Urge to push before complete cervical dilation: *(163)* _____

   _____

9. Explain the differences between these anesthesia professionals. *(164)*

    a. Anesthesiologist: _____

    _____

    b. Certified registered nurse anesthetist (CRNA): _____

    _____

10. Explain why it is usually best to avoid opioid narcotic analgesics if birth is anticipated within 1 hour of administration. *(165; Table 7-1)*

    _____

    _____

11. Describe the purpose for naloxone (Narcan), the patient most likely to receive the drug if needed, and the route(s) to administer the drug. Under what circumstances should naloxone not be given? *(165)*

    _____

    _____

12. For each type of regional anesthetic listed below, describe (i) how it is administered, (ii) the location of pain relief, (iii) its major side effects, and (iv) medical and nursing measures related to its use. *(See also Table 7-2)*

    a. Local infiltration *(167)*

        i.   _____

        _____

        ii. _____

        _____

        iii. _____

        _____

        iv. _____

        _____

    b. Pudendal block *(167)*

        i.   _____

        _____

        ii. _____

        _____

        iii. _____

        _____

        iv. _____

        _____

c. Epidural block *(167)*

   i. _____

   _____

   ii. _____

   _____

   iii. _____

   _____

   iv. _____

   _____

d. Subarachnoid block *(168)*

   i. _____

   _____

   ii. _____

   _____

   iii. _____

   _____

   iv. _____

   _____

13. An anesthesiologist often gives a test dose of the anesthetic agent when starting an epidural block to identify inadvertent injection into the _____ _____. The expected reaction to the test dose is _____. *(167)*

14. The woman who plans to have epidural anesthesia during labor and birth should be particularly questioned about allergy to _____ drugs. Why? _____
_____ *(167, Table 7-2)*

15. What is potentially the most life-threatening complication of general anesthesia for the mother? What is done to reduce the risk? *(169; Table 7-2)*

_____

_____

16. A woman receives an epidural narcotic after a cesarean birth. What should the nurse expect to assess related to this drug and for how long? *(172, Safety Alert)*

_____

REVIEW QUESTIONS

1. According to the gate control theory, which technique should be most helpful in interrupting transmission of labor pain to the brain? *(159)*
    1. Rapid, shallow breathing
    2. Application of heat
    3. Focusing on a point in the room
    4. Deep, cleansing breaths

2. Choose the best method during the admission process to help relieve general anxiety for a woman who has not attended prepared childbirth classes and who is having her first baby. *(162)*
    1. Assure her that she will be given pain medication any time she needs it.
    2. Determine her reasons for not attending the classes offered in the hospital.
    3. Have her take deep breaths to relax all muscles before doing any admission assessments.
    4. Give simple explanations about her environment and what to expect during labor.

3. Butorphanol differs from meperidine in that butorphanol: *(165; Table 7-1)*
    1. should not be used if a woman is dependent on heroin.
    2. causes greater respiratory depression in the newborn.
    3. better reduces the pain of late labor.
    4. cannot be reversed with naloxone.

4. The newborn of a woman who receives narcotic analgesics during labor should be observed primarily for: *(165; Table 7-1)*
    1. convulsions.
    2. slow respirations.
    3. excess activity.
    4. constipation.

5. An advantage of an epidural block is that it: *(166; Table 7-2)*
    1. reduces pain for both labor and birth.
    2. has no fetal or maternal risks.
    3. supports normal blood pressure.
    4. enhances the woman's urge to push.

6. Immediately after birth, nursing care for the woman who had subarachnoid block anesthesia for a repeat cesarean birth should include: *(172)*
    1. ambulating within 2 hours of birth.
    2. keeping her back curved outward.
    3. assessing for return of sensation.
    4. keeping her flat in bed for 8 hours.

7. A blood patch may be done to relieve: *(169)*
    1. low blood pressure.
    2. respiratory depression.
    3. postspinal headache.
    4. prolonged numbness.

8. The nurse should observe the woman who received epidural opioid narcotics for: *(165)*
    1. late respiratory depression.
    2. nausea and vomiting.
    3. unstable blood pressure.
    4. persistent headache.

9. During general anesthesia, cricoid pressure is applied to: *(166; Table 7-2)*
    1. reduce stomach acid secretion.
    2. avoid aspiration of gastric contents.
    3. prevent excessive blood loss.
    4. limit musculoskeletal injuries.

10. A pregnant woman asks if she should take prepared childbirth classes. The best response of the nurse is to tell her that classes will: *(158)*
    1. allow her to avoid pain medications during labor.
    2. be required if her partner wants to be with her.
    3. provide methods to help her cope with labor.
    4. reduce the likelihood that complications will occur.

11. The prepared childbirth technique that is most likely to relieve back pain during labor is: *(160, Box 7-1)*
    1. effleurage.
    2. sacral pressure.
    3. thermal stimulation.
    4. patterned breathing.

12. A woman is using prepared childbirth breathing techniques and complains of dizziness and tingling. The nurse should: *(164; Box 7-2)*
    1. have her breathe more rapidly with contractions.
    2. ask her if she feels an urge to push or bear down.
    3. tell her to exhale slowly into her cupped hands.
    4. reassure her that these sensations are normal.

13. Immediately after an epidural block is begun, the woman may be positioned: *(171; Nursing Care Plan 7-1)*
    1. flat on her back, with no pillow.
    2. upright with her legs over the side of the bed.
    3. with a small roll under her right hip.
    4. in a head-dependent position for block initiation.

14. Two hours after a vaginal birth with an epidural anesthesia, the nurse determines that the woman's bladder is full. The most appropriate initial nursing action is to: *(166, Table 7-2; 171, Nursing Care Plan 7-1)*
    1. help her walk to the bathroom if movement and sensation have returned.
    2. ask her how full her bladder feels before allowing her to walk to the bathroom.
    3. insert an indwelling catheter until the woman is at least 8 hours postpartum.
    4. take no action unless the woman says her full bladder makes her uncomfortable.

15. The most effective way to identify adequate maternal oxygenation after epidural administration of a narcotic for cesarean birth is to: *(172)*
    1. take the blood pressure regularly.
    2. observe for cyanosis or restlessness.
    3. maintain a side-lying position.
    4. observe pulse oximeter readings.

CASE STUDIES

1. Jill is a primigravida in labor at 4 cm cervical dilation. She is using breathing techniques she learned in prepared childbirth classes and is breathing rapidly throughout each contraction. She complains of stiff fingers and numbness around her mouth.
   a. What is the probable cause of Jill's symptoms?
   b. What is an appropriate nursing measure to help correct her problem?
   c. Jill is now 5–6 cm dilated and requests an epidural block. Is this an appropriate time during labor to give an epidural block? If so, what nursing observations are most important before and after the block is begun?
   d. What nursing measures are appropriate for Jill during the second stage of labor?

2. You are working with a laboring woman and note that she is holding her body stiffly and gripping the bed rails tightly during each contraction. What nursing interventions are appropriate in each of the following areas?
   a. Relaxation techniques
   b. Adjusting the environment
   c. Assisting her with breathing techniques

THINKING CRITICALLY

1. Why do you think general anesthesia is seldom used for vaginal delivery in the United States or Canada?

2. A woman who is 2 hours postpartum after an uncomplicated birth wants to go to the bathroom to urinate. She had an epidural block for pain relief during labor and the medication and catheter for the block were removed immediately after birth. The infant has been nursing at intervals and the mother has eaten a light meal.
   a. Should you allow her to use the bathroom or have her use a bedpan? Explain the reason for your choice.
   b. If you allow her to walk to the bathroom, describe what you should do to ensure her safety.

APPLYING KNOWLEDGE

1. When you are in the hospital, look at trays used to administer various anesthetics. Identify the following components on the trays.
   a. Pudendal block tray: trumpet
   b. Epidural block tray: Touhy or other needle used to insert into the epidural space, epidural catheter, and sizes of the needles and catheter in the tray
   c. Subarachnoid (spinal) block tray: spinal needle (note any size difference from the epidural needle)

2. Identify professionals in your hospital who administer obstetric anesthesia.
   a. Are they limited to administering specific types of anesthesia?
   b. Is one of these professionals present 24 hours a day?
   c. Do obstetricians give epidural blocks?

3. Discuss interventions of health professionals for women during labor with your classmates.
   a. What did you observe that reduced the woman's anxiety and pain?
   b. What increased anxiety and pain and was it possible to change these outcomes?

4. Look at the contents of emergency carts for women and newborns.
    a. Who usually handles emergency care of newborns who are in distress?
    b. Do they hold certification from the American Heart Association and American Academy of Pediatrics in neonatal resuscitation (NRP)?
    c. Which professionals are present at uncomplicated births or cesarean births to care for the infant?

5. What is the most common anesthesia for vaginal birth in your hospital? For cesarean birth?

6. Observe a laboring woman using childbirth preparation techniques.
    a. Who is her support person?
    b. How is the support person helping her use these techniques?
    c. How can you help her?

Nursing Care of Women with Complications During Labor and Birth

chapter

8

Answer Key: A complete answer key can be found on the Student Evolve website.

LEARNING ACTIVITIES

1. Match the terms in the left column with their definitions on the right (a–h).

   _____ Amniotomy *(176)*

   _____ Cephalopelvic disproportion *(181)*

   _____ Chignon *(181)*

   _____ Chorioamnionitis *(192)*

   _____ Dystocia *(183)*

   _____ Hydramnios *(184)*

   _____ Laminaria *(176)*

   _____ Macrosomia *(187)*

   a. Infection of the amniotic sac
   b. Excessive amniotic fluid
   c. Substance that swells within the cervix, dilating it slightly
   d. Circular swelling on the neonate's head caused by vacuum extractor
   e. Large body size
   f. Artificial rupture of the amniotic sac
   g. Inability of the fetus to fit through the pelvis
   h. Difficult labor

2. Describe three potential complications of amniotomy and the nursing assessments that should be done and recorded for each. *(176)*

   a. _____

   _____

   b. _____

   _____

   c. _____

   _____

3. Distinguish between labor *induction* and labor *augmentation*. *(174)* _____

   _____

   _____

4. Identify each drug or class of drugs from the following descriptions of their main purpose. Give examples of specific drugs for c and d.

   a. Soften the cervix: *(175)* _____

   _____

   b. Stimulate labor contractions: *(175-176)* _____

   _____

   c. Inhibit uterine contractions: *(175)* _____

   _____

   d. Speed fetal lung maturation: *(193)* _____

   _____

5. Describe three nursing measures to promote comfort in a woman who has an episiotomy or perineal laceration. *(180)*

   a. _____

   b. _____

   c. _____

6. What are the two separate incisions done in cesarean delivery? Which of the two is more important and why? *(182)*

   _____

   _____

7. What nursing observations are appropriate after cesarean birth in each of the following areas and why? *(183)*

   a. Vital signs and other types of monitoring:_____

   _____

   b. IV infusion: _____

   _____

   c. Uterine fundus: _____

   _____

   d. Dressing: _____

   _____

   e. Lochia: _____

   _____

   f. Indwelling catheter:_____

   _____

8. Compare *hypertonic* labor to *hypotonic* labor for the following characteristics. Note which one is most common. *(187, Table 8-2)*

Characteristic	Hypertonic Labor	Hypotonic Labor
a. Contractions		
b. Time of occurrence during labor		
c. Medical management		
d. Nursing care		

9. Describe how each of the following factors can contribute to abnormal labor and list nursing measures appropriate for each.

a. Ineffective pushing efforts: *(187)* _____

_____

_____

_____

b. Occiput posterior fetal position: *(189)* _____

_____

_____

_____

10. State five ways that excessive psychological stress can contribute to a difficult labor. *(191)*

    a. _____

    b. _____

    c. _____

    d. _____

    e. _____

11. Describe possible adverse effects of prolonged labor on either the mother or the fetus. *(191)*

    a. _____

    b. _____

    c. _____

    d. _____

    e. _____

12. Describe possible adverse effects of precipitous labor on the mother and fetus. *(191-192)*

    a. _____

    b. _____

    c. _____

13. a. What is the difference between PROM and PPROM? *(192)* _____

    _____

    _____

    _____

    _____

    b. How does your clinical facility test to see whether a woman's membranes have or have not ruptured? Does it ever test by looking at possible amniotic fluid under a microscope? If so, what does the midwife or physician see if the membranes have ruptured?

    _____

    _____

    _____

    c. Does a woman need this test if fluid is obviously leaking from her vagina? _____

    d. If a woman's membranes are ruptured, is there any difference in how she would be treated at 39 weeks gestation versus 29 weeks gestation?

    _____

    _____

    _____

14. What is the role of each of the following measures in the care of the woman with threatened or actual preterm labor? *(193)*

    a. Transvaginal ultrasound: _____

    _____

    b. Activity restrictions: _____

    _____

    c. Fetal fibronectin: _____

    _____

15. Describe five or more symptoms of preterm labor that should be taught to every pregnant woman. List additional symptoms that you or a friend experienced if preterm labor occurred. *(193)*

    _____

    _____

    _____

    _____

16. Describe nursing care of the fetus or neonate related to these problems of prolonged pregnancy. *(194)*

    a. Placental blood supply:_____

    _____

    b. Passage of meconium in utero: _____

    _____

    c. Consumption of glucose reserves prior to birth: _____

    _____

17. Describe four situations in which the nurse must be especially watchful for a prolapsed umbilical cord. *(194)*

    a. _____

    b. _____

    c. _____

    d. _____

18. List and describe three variations of uterine rupture. *(195)*

    a. _____

    _____

    b. _____

    _____

    c. _____

    _____

REVIEW QUESTIONS

1. After amniotomy, which observation should be reported immediately? *(176)*
   1. Clear fluid draining on the underpad
   2. Maternal temperature of 37.2° C (99.0° F)
   3. Fetal heart rate of 95 bpm
   4. Moderate contractions every 3 minutes

2. Which is the most appropriate nursing care for the woman having hypertonic labor? *(187, Table 8-2)*
   1. Encourage walking in the hallway to improve contractions and enhance labor.
   2. Promote rest and provide general comfort measures.
   3. Reassure her that this problem will go away when active labor begins.
   4. Omit oral fluids and increase the rate of intravenous fluid.

3. A woman—gravida 4, para 3—has been 5 cm dilated for 2 hours. Her contractions are every 7 minutes, 30 seconds duration, and mild. The FHR is 135–145/minute. She is relatively comfortable. This woman is most likely experiencing: *(187, Table 8-2)*
   1. hypotonic labor dysfunction.
   2. hypertonic labor dysfunction.
   3. occiput posterior fetal position.
   4. fetal shoulder dystocia.

4. After a vaginal birth complicated by shoulder dystocia, the nurse should particularly assess the newborn for: *(189)*
   1. molding of the head.
   2. flexed positioning.
   3. clavicle fracture.
   4. abnormal temperature.

5. A woman has ruptured membranes at 31 weeks gestation. Which nursing observation should be promptly reported? *(188, Nursing Care Plan 8-2)*
   1. FHR: accelerations present; average rate of 145 bpm
   2. Small quantity of clear, nonirritating vaginal discharge
   3. Spontaneous fetal movement with uterine palpation
   4. Maternal vital signs: T 38.2° C (100.7° F), P 102, R 20

6. Which is the most typical labor characteristic when the fetus is in an occiput posterior position? *(189)*
   1. Labor length under 3 hours
   2. Persistent back discomfort
   3. Rapid fetal descent
   4. Mild contraction strength

7. A woman who is at 32 weeks gestation telephones the nurse in a labor unit and says that her baby seems to be "pushing down" much of the time and that she has a constant backache. Choose the most appropriate nursing response. *(192)*
   1. Ask her to have someone bring her to the labor unit for further assessment.
   2. Reassure her that pressure and backache are common during late pregnancy.
   3. Tell her she should rest with her feet elevated several times each day.
   4. Encourage her to promote bladder emptying by increasing her fluid intake.

8. External version is most likely to be done in which of these situations? *(178)*
   1. Early labor with frank breech presentation
   2. Breech presentation with placenta previa
   3. Twins in cephalic and breech presentations
   4. Breech presentation at 38 weeks gestation

9. The first nursing action if a visibly prolapsed umbilical cord occurs is to: *(195)*
    1. call the physician or nurse-midwife.
    2. palpate the cord for a pulse.
    3. apply the internal fetal monitor.
    4. relieve pressure on the cord.

10. What is the priority nursing action following amniotomy? *(176)*
    1. Turn the woman to her side.
    2. Check the fetal heart rate.
    3. Assess the color of the fluid.
    4. Change the underpad.

11. The nursing intervention most likely to make the woman with a perineal laceration more comfortable during the first 2 hours after birth is: *(180)*
    1. warm-water soaks.
    2. a small dressing.
    3. an ice pack.
    4. antibacterial ointment.

12. Parents of a newborn delivered with low forceps ask about small bruises on each side of the baby's head. The nurse should tell the parents that the bruises: *(181)*
    1. will be reported to the physician.
    2. usually disappear in a few days.
    3. may indicate brain damage.
    4. occur in all vertex births.

13. Of the following options for cesarean birth, the most important nursing care during the postanesthesia recovery is to: *(186; Nursing Care Plan 8-1)*
    1. provide analgesia.
    2. assess the fundus.
    3. position for comfort.
    4. encourage urination.

14. When caring for a woman following a vehicle accident at 36 weeks of pregnancy, the priority fetal assessment should be for: *(196)*
    1. undetected trauma.
    2. poor oxygenation.
    3. intrauterine infection.
    4. precipitous birth.

15. The nurse must particularly observe for signs and symptoms of uterine rupture if the laboring woman just admitted at 8 cm has: *(195)*
    1. a hypotonic labor pattern.
    2. estimated fetal weight of 3500 g.
    3. prematurely ruptured membranes.
    4. a prior cesarean birth.

16. An infant's amniotic fluid was meconium-stained. During the admission assessment, the nurse notes that the infant is crying vigorously. Her skin is peeling and she has a long, thin appearance. These facts suggest that this infant is probably: *(194)*
    1. preterm.
    2. postterm.
    3. in respiratory distress.
    4. large for her gestational age.

17. A woman has a prostaglandin vaginal insert placed the day before she is scheduled for induction of labor at 40 weeks. Which is the most appropriate teaching immediately after the procedure? *(175)*
    1. "We will check your baby's heart rate after you walk for 30 minutes."
    2. "Expect vigorous and frequent contractions in about 30 minutes."
    3. "Call your nurse if you notice fluid leaking from your vagina."
    4. "Stay in bed on your left side until oxytocin infusion is started."

CASE STUDIES

1. Cara, a 24-year-old gravida 2, para 1, is in early labor with her second baby. Her cervix is 3 cm dilated and 75% effaced; fetal station is 0. Contractions are every 4 minutes, 30–35 seconds in duration, and of moderate intensity. The nurse-midwife performs an amniotomy. A small amount of light-green fluid drains on the underpad.
   a. Use your birth facility's standard form as a worksheet to chart this information about Cara's labor. If the facility charts with a computer, write in the information that would be documented on computer.
   b. Is the color of the amniotic fluid significant?
   c. What nursing interventions are appropriate specific to the situation above? Would other care providers in your facility be notified of these findings? List any providers who would be notified.
   d. Describe observations that would suggest that the amniotomy caused complications of any kind.
   e. If Cara's baby boy were born in a forceps-assisted birth, what observations should the nurse make in each area listed below? What observations would be significant in terms of complications?
      i.   Skin
      ii. Shape of head
      iii. Appearance when crying
   f. Write a simple explanation to parents about the appearance of the infant's head if his birth was assisted with a vacuum extractor.

2. Jennifer, a 32-year-old, is in spontaneous labor at term gestation of 39 weeks. Eight weeks ago, she was in a motor vehicle accident. She had a mild head injury and has recovered well. Greatest trauma occurred in her lower body, and includes fracture of her left pelvis and left femur. Jennifer remains in a long leg cast at labor onset. She needs an indwelling catheter for urine drainage related to epidural block analgesic and the needed infusion of large quantities of IV fluid.
   a. How can you adapt insertion of the indwelling catheter to maintain sterile technique?
   b. Describe how you used critical thinking to modify the standard catheter insertion technique for a person with no impairments.
   c. What problem(s) did you solve?
   d. How will your solution help prevent additional problems for Jennifer?

THINKING CRITICALLY

1. In addition to assessing the progress of labor, what other nursing assessments are important for the woman who has a precipitous labor? How can positioning the woman on her side improve the fetal oxygen supply?

APPLYING KNOWLEDGE

1. Observe newborns who were in abnormal presentations or positions before birth. Identify characteristics caused by the abnormal presentation or position. Was the method of delivery vaginal (spontaneous or assisted by vacuum extractor or forceps) or cesarean? If cesarean birth, was it scheduled?

2. What nursing interventions do nurses in your clinical setting use when a mother is having complicated labor? How did you contribute to a mother's physical or psychological comfort during labor? What was the reason for the woman's abnormal labor?

3. What drugs to stop preterm labor are prescribed in your clinical setting? Read the policies and procedures related to administration of the drugs for this purpose. If possible, assist in the care of a woman who is receiving the drugs. What concerns do the woman and her family express? If preterm labor contractions stop, does the woman remain in the hospital or is she discharged?

4. Make a list of activities appropriate for a woman on activity restriction for preterm labor, both in the hospital and at home. If available, discuss other therapies that may be offered to a woman with restrictions, such as physical, occupational, or recreational therapy, massage therapy, aromatherapy, or other complementary and alternative therapies.

5. How does your clinical facility determine if a woman's membranes have ruptured? Would additional tests be done if she is at 30 weeks gestation? Why?

6. Observe a woman who has a cesarean birth after labor, focusing on her feelings about the surgical birth. Compare your observations with those of classmates who have cared for other women who had scheduled cesarean births.

The Family After Birth

chapter

9

Answer Key: A complete answer key can be found on the Student Evolve website.

LEARNING ACTIVITIES

1. Describe the following expected assessments for the uterine fundus immediately after birth. *(205, Table 9-1, Nursing Tip)*

   a. Location: _____

   b. Consistency: _____

2. Describe the initial nursing action if the fundus is boggy (soft) and bleeding is excessive during the postpartum period. How does this action control uterine bleeding? *(202)*

   _____

   _____

3. List two drugs that may be ordered to correct a soft uterus and the acceptable routes of administration. Does your facility use other drugs for more severe bleeding? *(203)*

   a. _____

   b. _____

4. List and describe the three stages of lochia, including approximate duration of each. *(201, Skill 9-1)*

   a. _____

   _____

   b. _____

   _____

   c. _____

   _____

5. When should perineal care be done? *(204)*

   a. _____

   b. _____

6. What should the nurse teach a postpartum woman about doing perineal care and about applying and removing her perineal pad? Why is it important to do these procedures in this way? *(206, Skill 9-5)*

_____

_____

7. a. The new mother can expect her menstrual periods to resume in _____ weeks if she is not breastfeeding. *(205)*

   b. In the breastfeeding mother, return of ovulation and menstruation are _____. *(205)*

8. Average blood loss at birth is about _____ for vaginal birth and _____ for cesarean birth. *(205)*

9. Describe two nursing actions that may make a woman who is chilled and shaking after birth more comfortable. *(207)*

   a. _____

   b. _____

10. Describe two possible signs of a full bladder in the immediate postpartum period. *(201, Fig. 9-2)*

    a. Height of uterus: _____

    b. Location of uterus: _____

11. Describe five nursing actions to help a new mother empty her bladder after birth. Describe additional actions that you have found helped other patients (or you) empty the bladder more readily and completely. *(208)*

    a. _____

    b. _____

    c. _____

    d. _____

    e. _____

12. List three nursing measures to prevent or correct constipation after birth. *(208)*

    a. _____

    b. _____

    c. _____

13. Describe each of the following factors about postbirth use of $Rh_o(D)$ immune globulin (RhoGAM). *(209)*

    a. Mother's Rh factor: _____

    b. Infant's Rh factor: _____

    c. Recommended time of administration after birth: _____

    d. Site and route of administration: _____

14. Explain each of the following factors about postpartum rubella immunization. *(209)*

    a. Why it is given to the nonimmune woman at this time?_____

    _____

    b. Precautions: _____

    _____

    c. Safety during breastfeeding: _____

    _____

15. What assessments should the nurse make in each of these areas when caring for the woman who has had a cesarean birth? *(210; Nursing Care Plan 9-1)*

    a. Uterine fundus: _____

    _____

    b. Lochia: _____

    _____

    c. Dressing: _____

    _____

    d. Urinary output: _____

    _____

16. Name and describe Rubin's three postpartum psychological phases. *(211, Box 9-1)*

    a. _____

    _____

    b. _____

    _____

    c. _____

    _____

17. What are the appropriate nursing interventions for postpartum blues? *(212, Table 9-2)*

    _____

    _____

18. Describe nursing interventions that may be appropriate for grieving families in the maternity setting. If you wish, describe interventions that you or a family member or friend have experienced with grief, including grief other than infant loss. *(213-214)*

_____

_____

_____

_____

_____

19. Describe newborn behaviors during each phase of transition and the approximate duration of each stage. *(215)*

    a. First phase: _____

    _____

    b. Second phase: _____

    _____

    c. Third phase: _____

    _____

20. Why is prevention of neonatal hypothermia particularly important? *(215)* _____

    _____

    _____

21. How many arteries are in the newborn's umbilical cord? _____ How many veins? _____ What word can be used to help remember these numbers? _____ *(218)*

22. a. What is the minimum normal blood glucose on screening tests for a newborn (include units of measure)? _____ *(219)*

    b. List signs of hypoglycemia in a newborn. *(219)* _____

    _____

    _____

    _____

23. List seven common laboratory screening tests for newborns. Identify the one that is mandatory in all states. List additional newborn screening tests that are offered in your clinical facility and whether they are mandatory or optional. *(220)*

    a. _____

    b. _____

    c. _____

    d. _____

e. _____

f. _____

g. _____

Other: _____

24. List three types of parent-infant contact that enhance attachment. Which of these is most important? *(220-221; Fig. 9-7)*

    a. _____

    b. _____

    c. _____

25. a.   Describe colostrum. *(222)* _____

    _____

    b.   Explain the benefits of colostrum for the neonate. *(222)* _____

    _____

26. Describe methods to *prevent* and to *relieve* breast engorgement. *(224, Table 9-4; 228)* _____

    _____

    _____

    _____

27. Describe the following nutritional needs of the breastfeeding mother. *(230; see also Figure 4-7, p. 56)*

    a.   Calories:_____

    b.   Foods: _____

    c.   Fluids: _____

    d.   Supplements: _____

28. What should the nurse teach the breastfeeding mother in each of the following areas? *(230)*

    a.   Foods that the infant may not tolerate:_____

    _____

    b.   Medications: _____

    _____

29. List four types of infant formula. Give an example of the three main types. *(231)*

    a. _____

    b. _____

    c. _____

    d. _____

30. Describe the three common forms for infant formulas. *(231)*

    a. _____

    b. _____

    c. _____

31. Describe teaching in each of the following areas for bottle-feeding parents. *(232; Skill 9-7)*

    a. Propping the bottle: _____

    b. Size of nipple holes: _____

    c. Warming and microwaving: _____

    d. Burping: _____

    e. Positioning baby after feeding: _____

    f. Leftover formula: _____

32. Describe appropriate nursing teaching in the following areas for postpartum discharge. *(233)*

    a. Hygiene: _____

    _____

    b. Sexual intercourse: _____

    _____

    c. Diet: _____

    _____

33. List nine danger signals that a postpartum woman should promptly report to her physician or nurse midwife. *(233)*

    a. _____

    b. _____

    c. _____

    d. _____

    e. _____

    f. _____

    g. _____

    h. _____

    i. _____

34. Describe the following factors about automobile safety. *(233-234; Fig. 9-14)*

   a. Ideal position for infant: _____

   b. When a forward-facing seat can be used: _____

   c. Securing infant in seat and seat to vehicle: _____

   d. Airbag safety: _____

REVIEW QUESTIONS

1. Which postpartum patient assessment requires immediate nursing intervention? *(201, Nursing Tip)*
   1. Excretion of large amounts of urine on first postpartum day
   2. Soft uterine fundus, to right of the midline, 2 hours after birth
   3. Nipples intact but reddened on the first postpartum day
   4. Perineal area edematous with minor tenderness and slight bruising

2. The most serious potential problem if a woman's bladder is distended in the early postpartum period is: *(200, Fig. 9-2; 201)*
   1. infection.
   2. discomfort.
   3. vomiting.
   4. hemorrhage.

3. Which woman is most likely to have afterpains? *(201)*
   1. Gravida 1, para 1, 6.5 lb (2951 g) infant
   2. Gravida 3, para 1, 7 lb (3178 g) infant
   3. Gravida 1, para 1, twins weighing 3.5 lb (1589 g) and 4.5 lb (2043 g)
   4. Gravida 4, para 4, 9.5 lb (4313 g) infant

4. Two hours after a woman's uncomplicated vaginal birth requiring no anesthesia, the nurse notes that her uterus is firm, two fingerwidths above her umbilicus, and deviated slightly to her right side. The most appropriate nursing action at this time is to: *(202)*
   1. assess for shock or hemorrhage.
   2. massage her uterus continuously.
   3. insert an indwelling catheter.
   4. help her walk to the bathroom to urinate.

5. Choose the situation that describes appropriate administration of $Rh_o(D)$ immune globulin (RhoGAM). *(209)*
   1. Rh-negative infant, Rh-negative mother, given IV to the infant within 12 hours of birth
   2. Rh-positive infant, Rh-negative mother, given IV to the mother within 1 week of birth
   3. Rh-positive infant, Rh-negative mother, given IM to the mother within 72 hours of birth
   4. Rh-negative infant, Rh-positive mother, given IM to the mother within 72 hours of birth

6. When teaching parents about PKU testing, the nurse should teach them that: *(220)*
   1. a negative test indicates that their baby will not have brain damage.
   2. follow-up testing should be done during one of the early clinic visits.
   3. the test must be done before the infant nurses or has any formula.
   4. a special diet started with solid foods will prevent disability.

7. The nurse gives a postpartum woman a rubella immunization. Which is the most important patient teaching related to this immunization? *(209)*
   1. Neomycin can be used for rash or elevated temperature.
   2. Use a reliable birth control method for 3 months.
   3. Immunization now gives the baby immunity through breast milk.
   4. Increased urination is a common side effect of the immunization.

8. Colostrum's greatest benefit to the infant is prevention of: *(222)*
   1. constipation.
   2. weight loss.
   3. hemorrhage.
   4. infection.

9. The let-down reflex is stimulated by: *(223, 224; Table 9-4)*
   1. massage of the uterus.
   2. suckling of the baby.
   3. increased fluid intake.
   4. breast engorgement.

10. What should the nursing mother be taught about breast care? *(224, Table 9-4)*
    1. Clean the breasts with plain water when washing.
    2. Give one formula feeding daily to limit engorgement.
    3. Do not wear a bra the first few days after birth.
    4. Begin with the same breast at each feeding.

11. Parents should be taught that the safest position for their term newborn in the crib is: *(218, Nursing Tip)*
    1. with the head elevated.
    2. side-lying with head down.
    3. on either the back or side.
    4. prone with head elevated.

12. At her 2-week postpartum checkup, the woman's uterus should be: *(200)*
    1. two fingerwidths above the umbilicus.
    2. two fingerwidths below the umbilicus.
    3. just above the symphysis pubis.
    4. no longer palpable through the abdomen.

13. Diuresis in the early postpartum period indicates: *(207)*
    1. urinary tract infection.
    2. retention of body fluids.
    3. excretion of excess fluid.
    4. edema near the urinary meatus.

14. The earliest time when sexual intercourse can usually be resumed after birth is: *(233)*
    1. at 2 weeks postpartum.
    2. when a laceration heals.
    3. when lochia alba is present.
    4. after the 6-week check.

15. The most appropriate way to identify mother and infant when reuniting them is to: *(216, Fig. 9-5)*
    1. check the identification band numbers of each.
    2. ask the mother to clearly state her name.
    3. examine the mother's fingerprint and infant's footprints.
    4. verify that the names on the crib card and band are identical.

16. Which is the best nursing measure to increase the woman's perineal comfort during the first hour after vaginal birth with a midline episiotomy? *(204)*
    1. Help her take a warm sitz bath.
    2. Give her an oral analgesic drug.
    3. Apply topical anesthetic ointment.
    4. Place an ice pack on the area.

17. A mother phones the postpartum unit 4 days after birth. She says her baby cannot suck well on her nipples because her breasts are full and engorged. What should the nurse recommend? *(228)*
    1. Apply ice packs just before allowing the infant to nurse.
    2. Feed formula for the next two feedings to reduce pain and congestion.
    3. Massage the breasts and express a small amount of milk before nursing.
    4. Reduce daily liquid intake to 1 quart for a few days.

18. The nurse notes that a new mother has several bottles of partly consumed formula on her overbed table. Choose the most appropriate nursing action. *(232; Skill 9-7)*
    1. Recommend that she prepare bottles that contain only what the baby is likely to drink.
    2. Inform her that the bottles cannot be used because they have not been refrigerated.
    3. Tell her she may combine the leftover formula for the baby's next feeding.
    4. Check the room for other partially used bottles, then throw all of them in the trash.

19. Which lochia characteristic should the nurse teach the woman to report? *(233)*
    1. Change from red to pink-brown to white
    2. Cessation of flow by 4 weeks postpartum
    3. Return of red flow at 12 days postpartum
    4. Presence of a menstrual-like odor

CROSSWORD PUZZLE

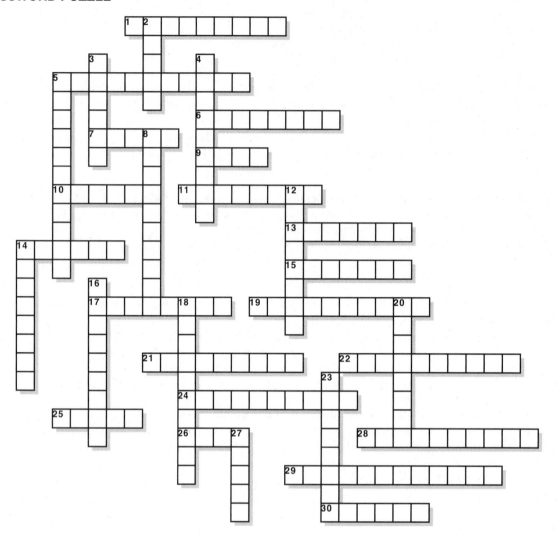

Across

1. Anterior pituitary hormone that stimulates breast to produce milk (223)
5. Heat loss caused when parent bathes infant slowly (215)
6. Giving or taking nourishment at the breast (225)
7. Vaginal folds (204)
9. Lochia that is mostly mucus (202)
10. Lochia that has a pink color (202)
11. Breast milk with higher fat content to satisfy infant's hunger (223)
13. Strong emotional tie that develops soon after birth (220)
14. Top of the uterus that contracts to control bleeding after birth (200)
15. Reflex that ejects milk from alveoli to the ductal system of nipple (223)
17. Posterior pituitary hormone that causes let-down reflex and uterine contractions (201, 203, 223) ·
19. Intermittent uterine contractions after birth; similar to menstrual cramps (201)
21. Heat loss caused by locating infant's crib near a cold wall (215)
22. Return of uterus to its normal state after birth (200)
24. Heat loss caused by air-conditioning vent blowing air on infant (215)
25. Brief feelings of joy and emotional letdown after birth (211)
26. Abbreviation for intrauterine growth restriction (217)
28. First 6 weeks after birth (199)
29. Milk secreted after colostrum (223)
30. Vaginal drainage that has three stages after birth (202)

Down

2. Bloody postpartum lochia *(202)*
3. Human milk having a bluish color *(223)*
4. Separation of the longitudinal abdominal muscles (rectus muscles) *(208)*
5. Father's intense interest in his new baby *(212)*
8. Long-term affection tie between the infant and parent *(220)*
12. Mood instability *(214)*
14. Watery, thirst-quenching breast milk *(223)*

16. First breast secretion; high in antibodies *(223)*
18. Heat loss caused when infant is placed on cool surface for assessment *(215)*
20. Drug used to reverse respiratory depression caused by epidural narcotics *(211)*
23. Good infant hold for breastfeeding woman who had cesarean birth *(224)*
27. Acronym used for assessment of episiotomy or other incision *(203)*

CASE STUDY

1. Cynthia, a 26-year-old, expects her first baby in about 12 weeks. She says that she is having a difficult time deciding whether to breastfeed or bottle-feed the baby.
   a. What information should you provide Cynthia to help her make this decision?
   b. What information would be available to use at your clinical facility?
   c. Cynthia decides to breastfeed her baby. On the fifth day after birth, she phones the unit to say that she has breast engorgement and her nipples are sore. Her left nipple has a small crack. What can the nurse teach Cynthia to help her cope with these problems?
   d. What should the nurse teach Cynthia about care of the baby's umbilical stump? What signs of problems should she report?

THINKING CRITICALLY

1. A woman has had a cesarean birth.
   a. What are some nursing interventions to help a mother manage pain while remaining alert enough to nurse her baby?
   b. Why is this mother likely to need additional nutrition teaching?
   c. What if her cesarean was done for placenta previa complicated by hemorrhage?

APPLYING KNOWLEDGE

1. What analgesics do postpartum women in your hospital receive for pain? Do nurses use any nonpharmacologic techniques to make the women more comfortable?

2. Observe families during the postpartum period.
   a. What interactions do you see among mother, father, and newborn?
   b. Identify practices in your clinical setting that enhance or inhibit parent-infant attachment.

3. Assist the staff nurse to help new mothers learn to breastfeed. If you have successfully breastfed a baby yourself, share appropriate helpful hints with new mothers and classmates.

4. Identify the protocol in your clinical facility for checking newborn glucose levels.
   a. Newborns who are routinely screened?
   b. Routine times for screening?
   c. Interventions for abnormal newborn glucose levels?

5. Role play with a classmate how to discuss the choice of breastfeeding or formula-feeding with a pregnant woman.

Nursing Care of Women with Complications After Birth

Answer Key: A complete answer key can be found on the Student Evolve website.

LEARNING ACTIVITIES

1. Match the terms in the left column with their definitions on the right (a–m).

   _____ "Baby blues" *(246, Nursing Tip)*

   _____ Bipolar disorder *(247)*

   _____ Curettage *(242)*

   _____ Postpartum depression *(247)*

   _____ Endometritis *(244, Table 10-2)*

   _____ Hematoma *(241)*

   _____ Homans' sign *(243)*

   _____ Hypovolemic shock *(238)*

   _____ Mania *(247)*

   _____ Mastitis *(246)*

   _____ Psychosis *(246)*

   _____ Pulmonary embolism *(243)*

   _____ Subinvolution *(242)*

   a. Infection of the uterine lining
   b. Infection of the breast
   c. Lodging of a blood clot in a blood vessel of the lung
   d. Calf pain when the foot is dorsiflexed
   e. Inadequate amount of blood to maintain normal circulation
   f. Mood disorder characterized by impairment of reality
   g. Mood disorder characterized by episodes of mania alternating with depression
   h. Hyperactive, excitable, euphoric behavior
   i. Delayed return of the uterus to its nonpregnant state
   j. Collection of blood within tissues
   k. Scraping or vacuuming the inner surface of the uterus
   l. Postpartum emotional state characterized by feelings of being let down, but generally satisfied with life
   m. Nonpsychosis characterized by loss of enjoyment, lack of interest, feelings of inadequacy after birth

2. Postpartum hemorrhage is blood loss that exceeds _____ mL after vaginal birth or _____ mL after cesarean birth. *(237)*

3. Early postpartum hemorrhage occurs within _____ hours of birth; late postpartum hemorrhage occurs later than _____ hours after birth until _____ weeks after birth. *(237)*

4. Describe the following five changes that occur in hypovolemic shock and indicate the change or changes that usually occur early. *(238-239, Nursing Care Plan 10-1)*

   a. Heart rate: _____

   b. Respiratory rate: _____

   c. Blood pressure: _____

   d. Skin and mucous membranes: _____

   e. Mental state: _____

5. Why does a poorly contracted uterus lead to hemorrhage? *(240)* _____

   _____

   _____

6. What is the connection between the infant suckling at the breast and control of postpartum bleeding? *(241)*

   _____

   _____

7. Describe typical differences in bleeding and uterine fundus characteristics between hemorrhage caused by uterine atony and that caused by a birth canal laceration. *(240; Table 10-1)*

   a. Bleeding

      i. Uterine atony: _____

         _____

      ii. Laceration: _____

         _____

   b. Uterine fundus

      i. Uterine atony: _____

         _____

      ii. Laceration: _____

         _____

8. Describe the following typical manifestations of a birth canal hematoma. *(241-242)*

   a. Visual appearance: _____

      _____

   b. Character of pain or pressure: _____

      _____

   c. Signs of blood loss: _____

      _____

9. How does manual removal of the placenta differ from the usual method of separation? *(242)*

_____

_____

10. Distinguish between the characteristics of a superficial vein thrombosis (SVT) and a deep vein thrombosis (DVT). *(243)*

    a. Superficial vein thrombosis:_____

    _____

    b. Deep vein thrombosis: _____

    _____

11. The greatest risk of deep vein thrombosis is that it may cause _____
    _____. *(243)*

12. Postpartum infection is generally characterized by a temperature of _____ after the first _____
    hours after birth, occurring on at least _____ days during the first _____ days after birth. *(244)*

13. List the localized signs and symptoms of an infection such as a wound infection. *(244; Table 10-2)*

    _____

    _____

14. Why are postpartum infections in the reproductive tract likely to spread? *(244)*_____

    _____

    _____

15. Why may the white blood cell (leukocyte) count be unreliable as the only assessment to diagnose infection after birth? *(244)*

    _____

    _____

16. What nutritional information is important when teaching the woman who has—or is at an increased risk of having—a postpartum infection? Would this teaching be appropriate for other people with an infection? *(244-245)*

    _____

    _____

17. Distinguish between *cystitis* and *pyelonephritis* in terms of the following characteristics. Which is the most serious? *(244; Table 10-2)*

    a. Fever:

        i.   Cystitis: _____

        ii. Pyelonephritis: _____

b.   Discomfort:

   i.   Cystitis: _____

   ii. Pyelonephritis: _____

c.   Other characteristics:

   i.   Cystitis: _____

   ii. Pyelonephritis: _____

18. Describe the following nursing measures to promote recovery from urinary tract infection and prevent future ones. *(245; Table 10-2)*

a.   Fluid intake: _____

_____

b.   Beneficial foods: _____

_____

19. Which two factors increase the likelihood that mastitis will develop? *(246, Figure 10-2)*

a.   _____

b.   _____

20. What is the role of heat application in the care of a woman with mastitis? *(244, Table 10-2)*

a.   _____

b.   _____

c.   _____

21. Describe three characteristics of subinvolution of the uterus. *(242)*

a.   _____

_____

b.   _____

_____

c.   _____

_____

22. Describe the basic difference between postpartum "blues" and postpartum depression. *(246-247)*

a.   Postpartum "blues": _____

_____

_____

b.   Postpartum depression: _____

_____

_____

REVIEW QUESTIONS

1. A woman had a forceps-assisted birth 2 hours ago. Baseline vital signs were T 37.1° C (98.8° F), P 78, R 20, BP 118/70. Which assessment suggests possible development of hypovolemic shock in this woman? *(238)*
   1. Firm fundus, slightly right of midline
   2. Pulse 100, respirations 24
   3. Respirations 22, blood pressure 114/76
   4. Light lochia rubra with small clots

2. A woman had a 16-hour labor that ended with the cesarean birth of a 4313 g (9.5 lb) infant. Her membranes were ruptured for 24 hours and oxytocin augmentation of labor was attempted before the cesarean birth. She has an IV infusion of Ringers' lactate and an indwelling catheter. For which complication should the nurse be most observant during the immediate recovery-room period? *(238-239; 240, Table 10-1)*
   1. Uterine atony
   2. Endometritis
   3. Uterine subinvolution
   4. Urinary tract infection

3. If the nurse finds that a new mother's uterus is soft, the appropriate initial action is to: *(241)*
   1. insert an indwelling catheter.
   2. massage the uterus until it is firm.
   3. check the woman's vital signs.
   4. increase the rate of the IV fluid.

4. One hour after vaginal birth, the nurse notes that a woman has a flat purple area, about 2 cm by 3 cm, on her perineum. Which is the most appropriate nursing action at this time? *(240; Table 10-1)*
   1. Assist her to take a warm sitz bath.
   2. Apply pressure with a tightly applied pad.
   3. Reapply a chemical cold pack on the area.
   4. Notify the physician of the observation.

5. When teaching a woman following vaginal birth 24 hours ago, the nurse should tell her to report: *(242)*
   1. pink vaginal drainage followed by red drainage.
   2. menstrual-like odor of vaginal discharge.
   3. uterine cramping when the infant nurses.
   4. excretion of large quantities of dilute urine.

6. Choose the most appropriate intervention to prevent deep vein thrombosis in a woman who is one day postcesarean birth. *(243)*
   1. Encourage her to walk several times each day.
   2. Provide her with increased fluids that she enjoys.
   3. Take her temperature to identify an elevation.
   4. Instruct her to stay in bed most of the day.

7. Choose the finding that suggests infection after birth. *(244, Table 10-2)*
   1. Poorly relieved perineal pain 4 hours postpartum
   2. Oral temperature of 37.7° C (100° F) 18 hours postpartum
   3. White blood cell count of 21,000/dL at 1 day postpartum
   4. Persistent and severe cramping 3 days postpartum

8. The best position for the woman who has postpartum endometritis is: *(244; Table 10-2)*
   1. semi-Fowler's.
   2. side-lying.
   3. supine.
   4. prone.

9. Which nursing assessment suggests that a postpartum woman has cystitis? *(244; Table 10-2)*
    1. Burning with every urination
    2. High fever accompanied by chills
    3. Fever with nausea and vomiting
    4. Voiding large amounts of urine

10. Which nurse's teaching is appropriate for the new mother who has cystitis? *(244; Table 10-2)*
    1. Eat several servings of whole grains and meats each day.
    2. Remain in bed except for going to the bathroom.
    3. Drink about 3 liters of noncaffeinated beverages daily.
    4. Take a stool softener to reduce added pain of constipation.

11. A woman is 8 hours postpartum after a spontaneous vaginal birth. Her admission hemoglobin was 9.5 g/dL, and her estimated blood loss during the birth was 1000 mL. She asks the nurse if she can walk to the bathroom. The best nursing response is to: *(243)*
    1. remind her that she should catch her urine in a "hat" to be measured.
    2. have her sit briefly on the side of the bed before helping her to the bathroom.
    3. encourage her to urinate every 2 hours to decrease the risk of excess bleeding.
    4. tell her to return to bed promptly after she finishes using the bathroom.

12. Which nursing assessment suggests infection of an episiotomy? *(244; Table 10-2)*
    1. Temperature of 37.8° C (100° F) 12 hours after birth
    2. Purplish discoloration of the perineum and labia
    3. Edema of the labia minora, labia majora, and perineum
    4. Redness of the perineum with separation of the suture line

13. A woman has postpartum uterine atony with hemorrhage. After bleeding is controlled, the physician orders an indwelling catheter mainly because it: *(239; Nursing Care Plan 10-1)*
    1. allows better estimation of the woman's fluid volume.
    2. identifies bloody urine that suggests bladder trauma.
    3. limits the need for the woman to ambulate to the bathroom.
    4. applies constant pressure against the bleeding uterus.

14. A woman who is 3 days postpartum comes to the emergency clinic because she is having pain and burning discomfort when she urinates. She denies that she has had any fever and states that her lochia is "light pink." The nurse should expect an initial order for: *(244, Table 10-2)*
    1. bladder analgesics.
    2. intravenous antibiotics.
    3. culture of vaginal discharge.
    4. clean-catch urine specimen.

15. A woman is 5 days postpartum and breastfeeding. She telephones the nurse at the clinic and says that her breasts feel very heavy and one of them is tender. She says the infant nurses "fair." The nurse should tell the woman that: *(244, Table 10-2)*
    1. her symptoms should go away when the infant begins nursing better.
    2. breastfeeding should be stopped until the pain goes away.
    3. a cold pack between feedings should reduce the pain.
    4. she should come to the clinic for evaluation of her symptoms.

16. Methylergonovine (Methergine) should be avoided if the woman has: *(241)*
    1. uterine atony.
    2. retained placenta.
    3. hypertension.
    4. endometritis.

17. Select the woman who is at greatest risk for bleeding from a vaginal wall laceration. *(240, Table 10-1)*
    1. Vaginal birth assisted with vacuum extractor
    2. First infant who weighs 3632 g (8 lb)
    3. History of uterine atony with previous birth
    4. Oxytocin (Pitocin) used to induce labor

18. Choose the foods that are highest in iron. *(246)*
    1. Citrus fruits, apricots, tomatoes
    2. Sweet and white potatoes, corn, dried beans
    3. Enriched bread, dark green leafy vegetables
    4. Milk, cheeses, legumes

19. A woman comes to the clinic for her 6-week postpartum check after having her first baby. She says to the nurse, "I don't know what's wrong with me. I'm exhausted all the time and yet I can't seem to sleep when I have the chance." The nurse should: *(246)*
    1. reassure her that the demands of being a mother can seem overwhelming, especially with the first baby.
    2. ask her if her partner, family members, or friends can help her with care of the baby and her home so she can rest.
    3. explain that women lose more blood at birth than they expect, and a slight anemia often leads to these symptoms.
    4. find a quiet place to talk with her about her feelings related to her new role as a mother.

20. Postpartum bipolar disorder is characterized by: *(247)*
    1. periods of letdown feelings but with general enjoyment of life.
    2. impaired reality characterized by euphoria alternating with depression.
    3. alternate periods of overeating and lack of interest in food and drink.
    4. prolonged feelings of worthlessness or guilt.

CASE STUDY

1. Carmen is transferred to the mother-baby unit after a cesarean delivery 2 hours ago following a long labor. Her healthy daughter weighs 4540 g (10 pounds). Carmen's blood loss during surgery was 1200 mL. Her vital signs on admission to the unit are: T 99° F, P 86, R 20, BP 118/80. Her fundus is firm, midline, and lochia is scant in amount. The dressing over her incision is clean and dry. The indwelling catheter bag contained 550 mL of light-yellow urine when it was emptied before transfer from the recovery room. Carmen is awake and says she is "really tired." She received epidural morphine (Duramorph) prior to leaving the operating room and rates her pain as 0 on a pain scale. (Use information from Chapters 7, 9, and 10 to answer the questions in this exercise.)
   a. Identify the priority nursing diagnosis for Carmen during her recovery period. What interventions are appropriate for this nursing diagnosis? What other important nursing diagnosis should be considered? Why?
   b. Carmen's vital signs are: T 98.6° F, P 96, R 20, BP 110/90 1 hour later. Lochia is moderate, with some small clots. Her catheter bag contains a very small amount of urine. She is slightly restless, but says she has no pain. How should you interpret these assessments? Do you need any other information? What action should you take?
   c. Are other complications more likely to develop later in the postpartum period? What do you think they would be based on this evidence?

THINKING CRITICALLY

1. How can the nurse's teaching about breastfeeding reduce the likelihood that a woman will develop mastitis? Give examples of what you might teach the mother of a term newborn.

2. A woman is having her 6-week examination after a normal vaginal birth at the office where you work. She has a "flat" appearance to her face and seems uninterested in what you say to her, although she cooperates with each request related to her examination and cares for her baby when he cries.
   a. What possibilities for her behavior should you consider?
   b. How should you respond to her?

APPLYING KNOWLEDGE

1. Look at the vital sign charts (including pulse oximetry if available) of several postpartum women.
   a. What is the pattern of their temperature and pulse rates after birth?
   b. Do you see any differences in these patterns among women who had a vaginal birth and those who had a cesarean birth?
   c. Can you see any effects of labor medication on vital signs?

2. Study the routine postpartum teaching given to all women before discharge. For each sign or symptom that a woman should report, identify the complications related to that sign or symptom.

3. Determine if your clinical facility provides written postpartum self-care instructions in languages other than English. If not, what provisions does the staff make for patients who do not speak English?

4. Ask if your clinical facility provides new mothers with information about postpartum depression. If provided, where is it documented? Watch an RN provide this information if possible.

The Nurse's Role in Women's Health Care

chapter

11

Answer Key: A complete answer key can be found on the Student Evolve website.

LEARNING ACTIVITIES

1. Match the terms in the left column with their definitions on the right (a–s).

_____ Basal temperature *(261)*

_____ Climacteric *(274)*

_____ Cystocele *(277)*

_____ Dyspareunia *(254)*

_____ Endometriosis *(254)*

_____ Hypospadias *(270)*

_____ Infertility *(269)*

_____ Libido *(274)*

_____ Menopause *(274)*

_____ Myoma *(272)*

_____ Osteoporosis *(274)*

_____ Pessary *(277)*

_____ Rectocele *(277)*

_____ Retrograde ejaculation *(270)*

_____ Spinnbarkeit *(261, Fig. 11-2)*

_____ Stress incontinence *(277; Nursing Care Plan 11-1)*

_____ Urge incontinence *(277)*

_____ Uterine prolapse *(277)*

_____ Varicocele *(270)*

a. Device inserted into vagina to support pelvic structures
b. Painful sexual intercourse
c. Presence of tissue resembling uterine lining outside the uterus
d. Release of semen into the male's bladder during sexual intercourse
e. Stretching of the cervical mucus at ovulation
f. Body temperature at rest, taken before any activity
g. Weak vaginal wall that cannot support the bladder properly
h. Weak posterior vaginal wall that inhibits proper stool passage
i. Inability to conceive when desired
j. Enlarged vein in the scrotum
k. Unexpected loss of urine when laughing, coughing, or sneezing
l. Inability to control urge to urinate due to overactive bladder
m. Cessation of menstruation
n. Benign tumors of the uterine muscle
o. Sexual desire
p. Period of time surrounding the cessation of menstruation
q. Loss of bone mass leading to bone fragility
r. Weakened support ligaments for the vagina and uterus
s. Urethral opening on underside of penis

2. a. The best time to perform breast self-examination is _____
   or _____. *(251; Skill 11-1)*

   b. Professional breast examination should be done _____ for all women over the age of
   _____. *(251)*

   c. The American Cancer Society recommends that mammography be done for all women aged _____
   at _____ intervals. *(251)*

3. List the preparation a woman should make before having a Pap test. *(251)*

   a. _____

   b. _____

4. a. The Pap test is recommended to start at age _____ years. *(253)*

   b. Every _____ years for women age _____ years. *(253)*

   c. Every _____years for women age _____ years. *(253)*

   d. No screening necessary *if* age ____>65 _____ years *and* _____ screening for the _____
   _____. *(253)*

5. Define each menstrual disorder below. *(253-254)*

   a. Amenorrhea:_____

   b. Primary amenorrhea: _____

   c. Secondary amenorrhea: _____

   d. Metrorrhagia: _____

   e. Menorrhagia: _____

   f. Mittelschmerz: _____

   g. Dysmenorrhea:_____

6. How can a low body weight contribute to amenorrhea? *(253)* _____

   _____

   _____

7. List common symptoms of premenstrual dysphoric disorder (PMDD). *(254)*

   a. _____

   b. _____

   c. _____

   d. _____

   e. _____

   f. _____

   g. _____

h. _____

i. _____

j. _____

k. _____

8. a. When do the symptoms of PMDD occur? *(254)* _____

_____

b. How many of the typical symptoms are required to diagnose PMDD? *(254)* _____

_____

c. Describe therapy that may be prescribed for PMDD. *(254)* _____

_____

d. Explain nursing responsibilities related to PMDD. *(254)* _____

_____

9. List four factors that contribute to vaginal infection and why they increase this risk. *(255)*

a. _____

b. _____

c. _____

d. _____

10. Describe important teaching related to toxic shock syndrome in each area listed. *(255; 256, Safety Alert)*

a. Handwashing: _____

_____

_____

b. Use of tampons: _____

_____

_____

c. Use of cervical cap or diaphragm for contraception: _____

_____

_____

11. a. Describe signs and symptoms of candidiasis. *(257; Table 11-1)* _____

_____

_____

b. List common medications used to treat candidiasis. *(247, Table 11-1)* _____

_____

_____

12. a. What is the most prevalent viral sexually transmitted infection (STI)? *(256; 257, Table 11-1)* _____

_____

b. What are the characteristics of this infection? *(256; 257, Table 11-1)* _____

_____

_____

c. What complications may occur during birth or after birth for the infant whose mother has this infection? *(259; Table 11-1)*

_____

_____

d. What malignant complication is associated with the infection and what precautions should the woman take related to this associated complication? *(259; Table 11-1)*

_____

_____

e. Visit www.cdc.gov/vaccines. Identify the following *current* facts about the vaccine for this viral STI. State the date that you retrieved this information from the CDC website and any other source(s) of information that you use to answer this question.

    i. Age recommended to begin vaccine series: _____

    ii. Number of shots needed and in what span of time: _____

    iii. Trade name or names of approved vaccines: _____

    iv. Estimated current cost: _____

13. How can chlamydia or gonorrhea infections result in infertility or an ectopic pregnancy? *(258; Table 11-1)*

_____

_____

14. a. The STI that has three possible stages is _____. *(258; Table 11-1)*

b. Describe the characteristics of each stage of this infection. *(258; Table 11-1)*

    i. Primary: _____

_____

    ii. Secondary: _____

_____

    iii. Tertiary: _____

_____

c.   What is the main drug used to treat it? Which alternate drug must be avoided during pregnancy? *(258; Table 11-1)*

_____

_____

15. Infections of _____ can reemerge later in outbreaks that are also infectious. *(259; Table 11-1)*

16. a.   Most oral contraceptives contain _____ and _____, while some contain only _____. *(262)*

b.   How does this drug or combination of drugs prevent pregnancy? *(262)* _____

_____

17. What is the significance of the ACHES acronym in relation to oral contraceptives? What does each letter stand for? *(263, Memory Jogger)*

A   _____

C   _____

H   _____

E   _____

S   _____

18. a.   Medroxyprogesterone acetate provides _____ months of effective contraception. It is given by the _____ route within _____ days of the menstrual period. *(263)*

b.   Why is this timing important? *(263)* _____

_____

19. List the three most common side effects of medroxyprogesterone acetate. *(264)*

a.   _____

b.   _____

c.   _____

20. What is the major difference among these intrauterine devices in terms of effectiveness? *(264)*

a.   Copper-containing (ParaGard): _____

b.   Levonorgestrel-releasing: _____

21. List two times when the diaphragm must be refitted. *(266)*

a.   _____

b.   _____

22. Describe appropriate teaching about condom use in each area listed. *(266; Skill 11-3)*

    a. Lubrication:_____

    _____

    b. Breakage or dislodgment during use:_____

    _____

    c. Expiration date: _____

    _____

    d. Removal: _____

    _____

23. Describe four methods that can be used for natural family planning. *(261)*

    a. _____

    _____

    b. _____

    _____

    c. _____

    _____

    d. _____

    _____

24. Why must another form of contraception be used for about 1 month following vasectomy? *(268)*

    _____

    _____

25. Describe two types of emergency contraception, including administration. *(267-268)*

    a. Oral contraceptives:_____

    _____

    b. Progestin only: _____

    _____

26. a. Define *primary infertility.* *(269)* _____

    _____

    b. Define *secondary infertility.* *(269)* _____

    _____

27. Describe the psychological reactions a couple may have to infertility. *(269-270)* _____

_____

_____

_____

_____

_____

28. a. Describe how each male factor can compromise fertility. *(270)*

    i.   Abnormal sperm: _____

_____

    ii. Abnormal erections: _____

_____

    iii. Abnormal ejaculation: _____

_____

    iv. Abnormal seminal fluid: _____

_____

  b. Describe how each female factor can compromise fertility. *(270-271)*

    i.   Disorders of ovulation: _____

_____

    ii. Abnormalities of fallopian tubes:_____

_____

    iii. Abnormalities of uterus, cervix, or ovaries: _____

_____

    iv. Hormone abnormalities: _____

_____

29. Describe similarities and differences among the following advanced reproductive techniques. *(273; Table 11-2)*

  a. In vitro fertilization (IVF): _____

_____

  b. Gamete intrafallopian transfer (GIFT):_____

_____

   c.   Tubal embryo transfer (TET): _____

        _____

   d.   Microsurgery: _____

        _____

30. Describe the following changes that may occur during the climacteric. *(274)*

   a.   Menstrual cycles: _____

        _____

   b.   Vasomotor instability: _____

        _____

   c.   Vaginal changes: _____

        _____

31. Describe changes in these structures that occur with loss of estrogen. *(274)*

   a.   Uterus and ovaries: _____

        _____

   b.   Vagina: _____

        _____

   c.   Pelvic musculature: _____

        _____

   d.   Bones: _____

        _____

32. a. Describe the advantages and risks of hormone replacement therapy (HRT). *(275)* _____

        _____

        _____

   b.   Explain conditions in which HRT is contraindicated. *(275)* _____

        _____

        _____

33. List six types of complementary therapy that may be used instead of, or as an alternative to, HRT and the purpose for each. *(275; Nursing Care Plan 11-1)*

   a.   _____

   b.   _____

   c.   _____

d. _____

e. _____

f. _____

34. Describe each variation of vaginal wall prolapse. *(277)*

a. Cystocele: _____

    _____

b. Rectocele:_____

    _____

35. What medical or surgical treatments may be used to reduce symptomatic uterine fibroids? *(278)*

    _____

    _____

    _____

    _____

REVIEW QUESTIONS

1. The nurse is teaching a woman, age 25, about breast self-examination (BSE). The correct teaching is that BSE: *(252; Skill 11-1)*
    1. detects malignancy more often than professional examinations.
    2. allows her to delay the need for mammography until she is 50 years old.
    3. helps her learn the normal characteristics of her own breasts.
    4. is more accurate than a yearly mammogram.

2. Choose the correct teaching about BSE technique. *(252; Skill 11-1)*
    1. Use the palms of the hand to press the breast tissue firmly against the ribs.
    2. Palpate each breast systematically, using the pads of the fingers.
    3. Palpate the underarm area only if the breasts are very large or sagging.
    4. Squeeze the breast tissue between the thumb and index finger.

3. Choose the correct teaching for relief of symptoms associated with premenstrual dysphoric disorder. *(254-255)*
    1. Eat chocolate candies several times a day to reduce fluid retention and weight gain.
    2. Reduce fluid intake during the first half of the menstrual cycle.
    3. Plan the most stressful activities during the last half of the menstrual cycle.
    4. Exercise individually or with others several times each week.

4. When teaching about the use of tampons, the nurse should emphasize replacing them at least every 4 hours to prevent: *(255)*
    1. pelvic inflammatory disease.
    2. vasomotor symptoms.
    3. sexually transmitted infections.
    4. toxic shock syndrome.

5. A friend asks you what she can do because she is troubled by repeated "yeast" infections. As a nurse, your best advice to her is to: *(257; Table 11-1)*
    1. keep over-the-counter medications on hand so she can begin treatment immediately.
    2. see her medical caregiver if she has another infection to identify possible causes.
    3. increase her intake of fluids to include at least eight glasses of water each day.
    4. avoid sexual intercourse for 1 month to see if that reduces the infections.

6. The long-term risk of an infection with the human papillomavirus is for: *(256)*
    1. cervical cancer.
    2. ectopic pregnancy.
    3. endometriosis.
    4. nerve damage.

7. Other than abstinence, the best way to prevent sexually transmitted infection with the human immuno-deficiency virus is: *(259, Table 11-1)*
    1. douching within 30 minutes of sexual intercourse.
    2. avoiding intercourse during midcycle.
    3. use of a condom for all episodes of sexual intercourse.
    4. taking prophylactic antibiotics after unprotected intercourse.

8. Choose the most appropriate teaching for the woman who is prescribed multiphasic oral contraceptive pills. *(262)*
    1. The menstrual period begins when the first week of pills is completed.
    2. Cigarette smoking should be limited to no more than 20 per day.
    3. Limit intake of foods that are high in iron or calcium.
    4. Take the pills at the same time of day and in order.

9. Choose the woman who should *not* take oral contraceptives. *(263)*
    1. A woman who has multiple sexual partners.
    2. A 38-year-old woman who smokes a pack of cigarettes daily.
    3. A 19-year-old woman who is formula-feeding her 2-month-old baby.
    4. A woman who is being discharged after a spontaneous abortion.

10. A woman has been taking oral contraceptives for 4 months. She is concerned because her periods are much lighter than before she started the pills. How should the nurse counsel this woman? *(262)*
    1. "You will probably have to stop the pill unless your periods become more like they were before."
    2. "We can switch you to a barrier contraceptive; your periods should return to normal in a few months."
    3. "Lighter periods are expected when you are on the pill, but you should tell us if they stop entirely."
    4. "Stop taking the pills immediately. We want to do a pregnancy test before you resume them."

11. Choose the correct patient teaching about the IUD. *(264)*
    1. "You should not use this contraception if you smoke or are over 35."
    2. "Check for the strings weekly for the first 4 weeks, then monthly."
    3. "Do not use tampons when you have your menstrual period."
    4. "Use another form of contraception for the first month after insertion."

12. Choose the contraceptive method from those listed that provides the best protection against sexually transmitted infections. *(266)*
    1. Female condom
    2. Hormone injection
    3. Intrauterine device
    4. Oral contraceptives

13. When teaching a woman the cervical mucus method to identify ovulation, the nurse teaches her that the normal character of the mucus near ovulation is: *(255)*
    1. thin and slippery.
    2. yellowish with a distinct odor.
    3. cloudy and sticky.
    4. thick, sticky, and clear.

14. Appropriate patient teaching following vasectomy is to: *(268-269)*
    1. apply heat to the operative area for 20 minutes at a time.
    2. abstain from intercourse for at least 6 weeks after the surgery.
    3. limit frequency of sexual intercourse for the first month.
    4. place an ice pack on the operative area to reduce discomfort.

15. A friend tells you that she is "having periods again." She thought she had her last menstrual period 2 years ago. As a nurse, you should advise her that she: *(275)*
    1. is probably having reactivation of estrogens that are causing the bleeding.
    2. should see a physician promptly because this is not an expected occurrence.
    3. should use a contraceptive if she does not want to become pregnant.
    4. probably has an infection of her vagina or cervix that should be treated.

16. "Hot flashes" are probably caused by: *(274; Nursing Care Plan 11-1)*
    1. anxiety about growing older and one's mortality.
    2. shifts in a woman's fluid and electrolyte balance.
    3. instability of the blood pressure.
    4. reduced estrogen secretion.

17. Choose the correct patient teaching about the drug alendronate (Fosamax). *(275)*
    1. Take food or milk within 30 minutes of the medication.
    2. Wash the nose out with saline 30 minutes after using the spray.
    3. Do not lie down for at least 30 minutes after taking the drug.
    4. Take calcium supplements at the same time as the medication.

18. Stress incontinence is best described as loss of urine: *(277)*
    1. during activities such as laughing or coughing.
    2. when in an anxiety-provoking situation.
    3. when vaginal infection occurs.
    4. during sexual intercourse.

19. What is the usual diagnostic procedure when an ovarian cyst is suspected? *(278)*
    1. Transvaginal ultrasound examination
    2. Bimanual pelvic examination
    3. Magnetic resonance imaging
    4. DNA and PCR testing

20. A nursing measure that can improve stress incontinence is to: *(278)*
    1. teach the woman to limit fluid intake to eight glasses of water each day.
    2. advise her to increase her fiber intake with raw vegetables and fruits and whole grains.
    3. encourage weight-bearing exercise at least three times each week.
    4. explain how and when to perform Kegel exercises.

CASE STUDY

1. Sharla tested positive for gonorrhea and chlamydia at her follow-up test 3 months after the previous infection for which she had treatment. She states that she took all her medicine and did not expect the infection to return. What teaching is appropriate to reinforce to Sharla about these two infections and their treatment? *(258; Table 11-1)*

THINKING CRITICALLY

1. When in clinical, note how many women are affected with hip fractures compared to the number of men affected.
    a. Does one ethnic group seem to be more affected than others?
    b. Do you notice signs of osteoporosis in these patients?
    c. What imaging techniques have been used to determine the location and severity of osteoporosis?
    d. Have you had a bone density scan?

APPLYING KNOWLEDGE

1. Interview nurses at a clinic about their experience caring for patients with STIs. Which diseases are most prevalent at this time in the local area?

2. Under supervision, teach a woman to perform BSE.

3. Observe a mammogram. Are multiple imaging techniques used to better evaluate breast tissue?

4. Visit www.cdc.gov/hpv/. What are the most current recommendations related to the human papillomavirus (HPV) vaccine?

The Term Newborn

Answer Key: A complete answer key can be found on the Student Evolve website.

LEARNING ACTIVITIES

1. Why does the United States require registration of all births and deaths in the neonatal and infant periods of life? *(281)*

   _____

   _____

   _____

2. Describe each reflex and state the age at which it is expected to disappear. *(282-283; 284, Table 12-1)*

Reflex	Description	Age at Disappearance
a. Moro		
b. Rooting		
c. Tonic neck		
d. Palmar grasp		

3. Normal newborn head circumference ranges from _____ inches to _____ inches or from _____ cm to _____ cm. *(283)*

4. List two functions of an infant's fontanelles. *(283)*

    a. _____

    _____

    b. _____

    _____

5. Describe the following characteristics of the anterior fontanelle. *(283; 285, Skill 12-1)*

    a. Shape: _____

    b. Location (bones): _____

    c. Time of closure: _____

6. Describe the following characteristics of the posterior fontanelle. *(283; 285, Skill 12-1)*

    a. Shape: _____

    b. Location (bones): _____

    c. Time of closure: _____

7. Describe the three steps for using a bulb suction to remove a newborn's excess secretions. *(288-289; Skill 12-2)*

    a. _____

    b. _____

    c. _____

8. Explain the two types of heart murmurs that can be heard in newborns. Indicate which may cause problems. *(289)*

    a. Functional: _____

    _____

    b. Organic: _____

    _____

9. a. What is a common route for taking a newborn's first temperature? *(290)* _____

    _____

    b. Subsequent temperatures are taken by what route? *(290)* _____

    _____

   c. What is the correct technique for taking the temperature by each method? *(290)*

      i. _____

      ii. _____

10. State normal ranges for each of these newborn vital signs and signs that the nurse should promptly report. *(290; Fig. 12-9)*

Vital Sign	Normal Range	Signs to Report (include both rate and character as appropriate)
a. Temperature (state both Fahrenheit and Centigrade)		
b. Pulse		
c. Respirations		

11. Give the average range for these newborn measurements. *(291)* _____

   a. Length _____ to _____ cm (_____ to _____ inches)

   b. Weight _____ to _____ g (_____ to _____ pounds)

12. Describe the following normal musculoskeletal assessments for a newborn, including possible deviations from normal. *(290-291)*

   a. Movements: _____

   b. Eyes:_____

   c. Tremors:_____

   d. Muscle tone: _____

13. Describe the following characteristics and functions of a newborn infant's kidneys. *(292)*

   a. Blood flow: _____

      _____

b. Reabsorption functions: _____

_____

c. Concentration of urine: _____

_____

d. Capacity to handle fluid imbalances: _____

_____

14. Expectant parents are attending a prepared childbirth class in which you discuss circumcision. Several ask you if their sons should have the procedure done and another couple said they thought all boys were circumcised. What should you tell these couples about the advantages and disadvantages of circumcision? What should you tell them about circumcision in the Jewish faith? *(292-293; Fig. 12-12; Patient Teaching: Home Care of the Penis)*

a. Advantages: _____

_____

b. Disadvantages: _____

_____

c. Circumcision in Jewish families: _____

_____

15. Explain each of the following aspects of circumcision care in a way you might teach parents. Describe how these interventions are done in your clinical facility. *(292-293)*

a. Pain relief that may be used: _____

_____

b. Comforting: _____

_____

c. Maintaining warmth: _____

_____

d. Bleeding: _____

_____

e. Urination: _____

_____

16. a. Explain the normal occurrences that cause physiologic jaundice. *(294)* _____

_____

_____

b. Physiologic jaundice appears at about _____ days after birth and lasts for about _____ week(s). *(294; Skill 12-4)*

17. Describe the following typical stools in the newborn, including the time they appear, if applicable. *(299; Fig. 12-15)*

    a. Meconium: _____

    _____

    b. Transitional stool:_____

    _____

    c. Stool of breastfed baby:_____

    _____

    d. Stool of formula-fed baby: _____

    _____

18. Describe three types of abnormal stools in the newborn. *(299)*

    a. _____

    b. _____

    c. _____

19. Describe stools in constipation. *(299)*_____

    _____

    _____

20. The newborn's stomach has a capacity of about _____ mL and empties in about _____ hours. *(300)*

21. Why is it important to prevent infection in a newborn and what characteristic of the newborn's response to infection can make it difficult to recognize? *(300)*

    _____

    _____

REVIEW QUESTIONS

1. Which reflex shows the baby's reaction to sudden movement by drawing up the legs, extending the arms, then folding the arms across the chest with the fingers open? *(282; 284, Table 12-1)*
   1. Dancing
   2. Moro
   3. Rooting
   4. Grasp

2. When teaching a mother how to nurse her baby, how should you explain the baby's rooting reflex? The rooting reflex: *(282)*
   1. shows equality of function on each side of the mouth.
   2. helps the baby keep mucus or milk from being inhaled during breathing.
   3. suggests that the baby is full as he or she turns away from the breast.
   4. is the baby's way of seeking her nipple to obtain milk when hungry.

3. In the birthing room, a first-time father asks the nurse why the baby's head is "long and pointy." The nurse should respond: *(283)*
    1. "The head changes shape so it can pass through the mother's pelvis during birth."
    2. "Fluid builds up within the head before and during birth; it will go away in a few days."
    3. "Labor causes slight bleeding into the space between the skull bones and their covering."
    4. "We will notify the pediatrician, who will probably order an MRI of the baby's head."

4. Visually, babies prefer: *(283)*
    1. geometric objects.
    2. soft or pastel colors.
    3. the human face.
    4. stationary objects.

5. The correct way to suction a baby's mouth with a bulb syringe is to: *(288, Skill 12-2)*
    1. compress the bulb, place the tip in the side of the mouth, then release the bulb.
    2. place the tip in the side of the mouth, compress the bulb, then release the bulb.
    3. compress the bulb, place the tip in the center of the mouth, then release the bulb.
    4. place the tip in the center of the mouth, compress the bulb, then release the bulb.

6. When admitted to the nursery, a baby's initial rectal temperature is 35.8° C (96.6° F). Choose the most appropriate nursing response for this assessment. *(289)*
    1. Chart the expected temperature and continue doing other admission assessments and measurements.
    2. Keep the baby in a radiant warmer during admission and recheck the temperature in 30 minutes.
    3. Remove blankets and sources of added heat from the baby.
    4. Recheck the temperature in 30 minutes to verify accuracy.

7. One hour after a Plastibell circumcision, the nurse notes a small amount of blood oozing from the area. Which is the appropriate initial nursing response to this observation? *(293)*
    1. Continue to observe for increased bleeding.
    2. Apply pressure with a gauze pad and gloved fingers.
    3. Call the physician who performed the procedure.
    4. Wrap petroleum jelly gauze around the penis.

8. A new mother asks why her 2-day-old baby's skin appears slightly yellow. Which is the best nursing response to explain the cause of this skin color? *(294; 295, Safety Alert)*
    1. Small blood vessels are broken during labor, releasing waste products into the blood.
    2. The baby's digestive tract is immature and cannot yet excrete bilirubin effectively.
    3. Skin color changes slightly during the first few weeks until the permanent color is evident.
    4. Excess blood cells are being broken down rapidly because the baby is now breathing air.

9. New parents should be taught to clean their baby's ears by: *(287)*
    1. moistening a cotton-tipped applicator with water and rotating it in the ear canal.
    2. gently instilling a small amount of warm water into the ear with a bulb syringe.
    3. applying baby oil to a rolled piece of cotton and inserting it into the ear.
    4. wiping the outside with a cotton ball that is moistened with water.

10. A small area of a 6-day-old term infant's abdominal skin remains distorted when pinched gently. This assessment suggests: *(294, Fig. 12-13)*
    1. poor hydration.
    2. postbirth edema.
    3. excessive intake of breast milk or formula.
    4. inadequate vernix during the prenatal period.

11. What should the parents be taught about caring for the umbilical cord? *(296, Skill 12-5)*
    1. Bathe the baby in a small basin to cleanse the cord on all surfaces.
    2. A sponge bath is easy and allows the cord to remain dry until healed.
    3. Use an oil-based cleanser to speed healing of the baby's cord site.
    4. Baths are not needed until the cord site has healed to reduce infection.

12. An infant has a small laceration on the forehead when delivered by cesarean. Brief finger pressure in the operating room stopped the bleeding and the physician does not need to suture the laceration. The nurse should primarily observe for what other complication related to the baby's laceration? *(300)*
    1. Anemia, possibly manifested by pallor and tachycardia
    2. Hypothermia due to delay of placement in a warmer
    3. Excessive erythrocyte destruction and early jaundice
    4. Infection limited to the site or possibly generalized

13. A newborn has a heelstick for studies. The mother is concerned because the baby is crying loudly. The best response of the nurse is: *(288)*
    1. "That's the only way the baby can communicate with us."
    2. "Hold the baby close and comfort him by gentle rocking."
    3. "Babies cannot feel pain because they are immature."
    4. "The baby will only cry for a few minutes at most."

14. How should the nurse respond to acrocyanosis in a 12-hour-old infant? *(290)*
    1. Administer oxygen through an infant-sized mask.
    2. Apply heat with an incubator or radiant warmer.
    3. Assess the pulse and respirations for abnormal rates.
    4. Continue routine newborn nursing observations.

15. Which is an abnormal clinical assessment for a Latino boy at 1 week of age? Birth weight was 3772 g (8 pounds, 5 ounces); vital signs at hospital discharge time were: T 36.8° C (98.4° F) (axillary); P 142; R 40. There were no complications during pregnancy. *(291-292)*
    1. The infant weighs 3318 g (7 pounds, 5 ounces).
    2. The apical pulse is 130 bpm and slightly irregular.
    3. The infant has bluish areas on the lower back.
    4. The infant has tiny, white, raised papules on the nose.

16. A new mother asks why her term newborn sometimes "shakes" when he cries. Choose the best nursing response. *(291)*
    1. "Why not ask the baby's doctor about this when she makes rounds?"
    2. "The baby is easily upset and waves his arms to show his irritation."
    3. "An infant's muscles are too weak to move steadily."
    4. "This is a normal newborn behavior during crying."

17. A term newborn should pass the first meconium stool no later than how many hours after birth? *(299)*
    1. 6
    2. 12
    3. 24
    4. 36

18. A new mother is concerned because her 3-day-old daughter has a slightly blood-tinged vaginal mucus discharge. How should the nurse respond to this mother's concern? *(293)*
    1. "The baby could have a minor abnormality in her vagina."
    2. "Has there been any kind of injury to this area?"
    3. "Effects of your pregnancy hormones cause this response."
    4. "This should be reported to the doctor right away."

19. The nurse should teach parents to avoid using baby powder because it: *(295)*
    1. irritates the newborn's respiratory tract.
    2. may cause allergies in the newborn.
    3. is difficult to remove during a bath.
    4. dries the skin of the axillae and groin.

20. An infant looks at her mother and remains quiet when the mother sings to her in soft, high-pitched tones. This is an example of: *(287)*
    1. a sign of impaired hearing.
    2. the quiet alert state of reactivity.
    3. a need for reduced stimulation.
    4. limited ability to respond to adults.

CROSSWORD PUZZLE

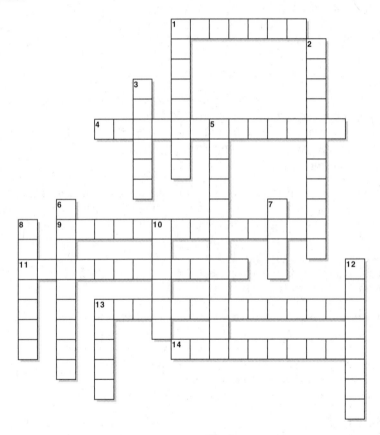

Across

1. Shaping of the head from pressure during birth *(283)*
4. Cheeselike substance covering newborn skin (two words) *(294)*
9. Collection of blood beneath the periosteum of the skull *(283)*
11. Bluish color of the hands and feet *(294)*
13. Bluish spots or discolorations of the skin, usually in dark-skinned babies (two words) *(294)*
14. Soft area at intersection of skull bones *(283)*

Down

1. First stool *(299)*
2. Urethral opening on the underside of penis *(292)*
3. Term used to describe tissue elasticity *(294)*
5. Removal of the foreskin of the penis *(292)*
6. Full-term infant's resistance to attempts to bring one elbow farther than the midline of the chest (two words) *(291)*

7. Name for reflex in which infants draw their legs up and the arms fan out and then come toward midline in an embrace position *(282)*
8. Newborn's inability to maintain neutral head position (two words) *(282)*

10. Fine hair covering the body *(294)*
12. White dots on the palate with the appearance of pearls *(294)*
13. Small, white, pinpoint bumps, usually on the nose or chin *(294)*

CASE STUDY

1. Jessica and Casey, a couple in their mid-20s, have a new son named Aiden who is now 16 hours old, weighs 7 pounds, 9 ounces, and is breastfeeding. Jessica wants to go home about 36 hours after birth. Aiden will be circumcised (Plastibell) before discharge. Jessica and Casey have no nearby relatives and are the first couple in their circle of friends to have a baby. They have read books on baby care but are concerned about actually caring for their baby's needs. The couple says they need to know "everything." (You are encouraged to use any of your facility's teaching materials as you complete this case study.)
   a. For each area listed, explain what content you will teach them.
      i. Safety
      ii. Using bulb syringe
      iii. Taking their baby's temperature
      iv. Maintaining an optimal body temperature
   b. How can you encourage the parents to participate in each topic so they will feel more secure?
   c. How will you incorporate information they may have read in books?
   d. Because Aiden will be discharged soon after being circumcised, what should you teach the parents about care and observation for complications? What actions may comfort him?

APPLYING KNOWLEDGE

1. Assist with admitting newborns and administer prophylactic eye care and vitamin K injections.
   a. What initial and ongoing cord care does your facility use and with what frequency?
   b. Does your facility offer the first hepatitis B immunization with newborn care?
   c. Do parents sign a consent form for any of these procedures? If so, which one(s)?

2. Does your facility use an instrument to check bilirubin levels in the newborn's skin? Describe how the nurse arrives at the most accurate bilirubin level with the instrument and how that level is documented and at what time intervals.

3. Observe newborns in the nursery for characteristics listed in the textbook.
   a. Distinguish between normal characteristics and those that may indicate a problem.
   b. What action is taken for deviations from normal?

4. Observe a circumcision.
   a. What type of circumcision is most common in your hospital?
   b. Observe newborns after circumcision for bleeding and urination.

5. Does your hospital have a standard infant care teaching plan for new parents? If so, what does the plan include? Observe how different staff nurses incorporate parent teaching into their care of mothers and babies. How have short stays influenced parent teaching?

6. A baby is coming to the office for a checkup at 1 week of age. He weighed 8 pounds, 6 ounces at birth. He now weighs 7 pounds, 7 ounces. Has the baby's weight loss been within normal limits or is it excessive? Justify your answer.

7. Log onto www.cdc.gov and locate birth data (natality data) from the alphabetic list of topics. This will give you the latest data to answer many specific questions and most of these are through National Center of Health Statistics. Here is content that the reader can usually find with this search.
   a. What is the newest *final* data on births that you find? What is the year of these births?
   b. How do you see trends for births at less than 39 weeks gestation? How does this compare to your clinical site?
   c. Find out the birth rate for your clinical facility during the past year. Pick a month and see if you can determine the gestation of each. Can you find how many babies were born full term (39 or more weeks)? Early term (37-38 weeks)? Late preterm (34-36 weeks)? Early preterm (<34 weeks)?
   d. Seek other information that looks interesting to you in this category.

Preterm and Postterm Newborns

Answer Key: A complete answer key can be found on the Student Evolve website.

LEARNING ACTIVITIES

1. Match the terms in the left column with their definitions on the right (a–p).

   _____ Apnea *(312)*
   _____ Ballard scoring system *(309, Fig. 13-2)*
   _____ Bradycardia *(312)*
   _____ Bronchopulmonary dysplasia *(312)*
   _____ Circadian rhythm *(320; Fig. 13-6)*
   _____ Gestational age *(320)*
   _____ Hypoglycemia *(309)*
   _____ Kangaroo care *(317)*
   _____ Kernicterus *(316)*
   _____ Neutral thermal environment *(316)*
   _____ Preterm infant *(309)*
   _____ Postterm infant *(309)*
   _____ Sepsis *(313)*
   _____ Surfactant *(311)*
   _____ Early term infant *(309)*
   _____ Total parenteral nutrition *(318)*

   a. Provision of full nutrition by the parenteral (IV) route
   b. Length of time spent in the uterus
   c. Cessation of breathing for 20 seconds or more
   d. Lung secretion that facilitates oxygen exchange
   e. Nervous system damage caused by high levels of bilirubin in the blood
   f. Method of estimating newborn maturity by physical and neurologic characteristics
   g. Heart rate lower than 100 bpm in the newborn
   h. Generalized infection
   i. Low blood glucose (blood sugar) level
   j. Control of temperature, air, surface temperature, and humidity to minimize an infant's oxygen consumption
   k. Born after less than 37 weeks gestation
   l. Born between 37 weeks and 38 weeks, 6 days
   m. Born after more than 42 weeks gestation
   n. Warming an infant by skin-to-skin contact
   o. Sleep pattern
   p. Condition that may cause an infant to have a prolonged dependence on a ventilator

2. Describe the following typical physical characteristics of a preterm infant's appearance. *(309)*

   a. Skin: _____

   b. Superficial veins: _____

   c. Subcutaneous fat:_____

   d. Lanugo: _____

   e. Vernix caseosa: _____

   f. Sole creases: _____

    g. Abdomen: _____

    h. Nails: _____

    i. Genitalia: _____

3. a. Respiratory distress syndrome (RDS) is associated with an inadequate quantity of
      _____ in the lungs. *(310-311)*

    b. At what gestational age is an infant expected to have an adequate quantity of this substance? *(312)*

    _____

    c. If an infant is born before the gestational age in question 3b, what is the usual therapy? *(312)*

    _____

4. If preterm birth appears inevitable, what drug for the mother should the nurse anticipate before birth? *(312)*

    _____

5. List two signs that may accompany apnea. *(312)*

    a. _____

    b. _____

6. List seven factors that make the preterm infant more vulnerable to loss of body heat than a term infant. *(314)*

    a. _____

    b. _____

    c. _____

    d. _____

    e. _____

    f. _____

    g. _____

7. a. Hypoglycemia in the infant is defined as a plasma level of glucose lower than _____ mg/dL in the term infant and _____ mg/dL in the preterm infant. *(314)*

    b. List two reasons why a preterm infant is prone to hypoglycemia. *(314)*

      i. _____

      ii. _____

    c. Describe preterm newborn conditions that are likely to increase the infant's need for more glucose. *(314)*

    _____

    _____

8. What two factors predispose a preterm infant to bleeding? *(315)*

   a. _____

   b. _____

9. Describe five factors that impair the preterm infant's nutritional function. *(315)*

   a. _____

   b. _____

   c. _____

   d. _____

   e. _____

10. a. What is the pathology of necrotizing enterocolitis (NEC)? *(315)* _____

    _____

    _____

    b. List signs that indicate an infant may have NEC. *(315)* _____

    _____

    _____

11. a. Pathologic jaundice may appear within _____ hours and/or may increase at a rate greater than _____ mg/dL in 24 hours. *(316)*

    b. Breast milk jaundice usually appears at _____ days and peaks _____ to _____ days after birth. *(316)*

    c. Explain why the infant with late breast milk jaundice may receive formula. How long is formula substituted for this infant? *(316)*

    _____

    _____

    _____

12. The ideal milk for the preterm infant is _____ milk. *(317)*

13. List three methods by which the preterm infant can receive nourishment. *(317-318)*

    a. _____

    b. _____

    c. _____

14. a. The two usual positions for the preterm infant are _____ or _____ _____. *(318)*

b. How do these positions differ from those recommended for a term infant with no respiratory problems? How will you explain this difference to parents? *(318, 320; see also Chapter 25, pp. 581, 583)*

_____

_____

15. List seven problems associated with caring for a postterm newborn. *(321)*

a. _____

b. _____

c. _____

d. _____

e. _____

f. _____

g. _____

16. Describe the following typical physical characteristics of the postterm newborn. *(321)*

a. General body appearance: _____

_____

b. Presence of lanugo: _____

_____

c. Presence of vernix caseosa:_____

_____

d. Skin appearance: _____

_____

REVIEW QUESTIONS

1. Which physical characteristic should make the nurse think an infant's gestational age may be preterm? *(309)*
    1. Square window sign assessed at 0 degrees.
    2. Small amount of lanugo and vernix present.
    3. Labia majora cover labia minora of the female.
    4. Superficial scalp and abdominal veins easily seen.

2. Gestational age is best determined by: *(309)*
    1. weight of the infant at birth.
    2. stability of the blood glucose level.
    3. the age at which the infant reaches developmental milestones.
    4. assessment of physical and neurologic characteristics.

3. A preterm infant is subject to hypothermia because the: *(316; 318, Nursing Care Plan 13-1)*
   1. muscle activity is large related to the calories consumed.
   2. relatively large body surface area allows heat to escape.
   3. sweat glands are overactive, allowing evaporative cooling.
   4. fat stores insulate the infant from radiant heater warmth.

4. Choose the normal blood glucose level for a preterm infant. *(314)*
   1. 28 mg/dL
   2. 39 mg/dL
   3. 55 mg/dL
   4. 150 mg/dL

5. The nurse must handle the preterm infant gently because capillaries are: *(315)*
   1. not developed in all areas of the brain.
   2. likely to develop microscopic clots.
   3. sensitive to high levels of clotting factors.
   4. fragile and prone to bleed spontaneously.

6. The advantage of radiant warmers in the care of preterm infants is that they: *(314)*
   1. cannot cause excessive body temperature.
   2. maintain warmth with easy caregiver access.
   3. reduce drying and cracking of the skin.
   4. improve balance of fluids and electrolytes.

7. The ideal feeding for most preterm newborns is: *(317; Nursing Care Plan 13-1, 318)*
   1. glucose water until the risk for necrotizing enterocolitis diminishes.
   2. breast milk given by suckling, bottle, or gavage.
   3. special commercial formula for preterm babies.
   4. total parenteral nutrition to meet all of the infant's nutritional needs.

8. An infant is brought to the newborn nursery. The gestation stated on the chart is 39 weeks. The nurse doing the initial assessment notes that the infant has peeling skin and a long, thin appearance. What is the probable reason for the infant's appearance? *(321)*
   1. The mother did not get adequate nutrients throughout pregnancy.
   2. Intrauterine infection depleted subcutaneous fat stores.
   3. The actual gestational age may be greater than 42 weeks.
   4. Reduced production of glucose before birth caused weight loss.

9. A mother gives birth to a preterm infant at 30 weeks gestation. When visiting the baby in the intensive care unit, she seems interested in the baby, but sits and watches everything the nurse does for her baby. Which is the most appropriate nursing intervention to promote mother-infant attachment? *(318; 320-321, Nursing Tip)*
   1. Invite her to provide simple care to her infant.
   2. Reassure her that she can hold the baby soon.
   3. Stress the importance of frequent visits to the nursery.
   4. Demonstrate the skills she will need for home care.

10. Which nursing assessment best suggests respiratory distress syndrome? *(311)*
    1. Apical heart rate 144/min; bluish hands and feet
    2. Grunting, respiratory rate of 65/min, nasal flaring
    3. Protruding abdomen, irregular respirations
    4. Weak movements, lies with extended posture

11. The alarm on an apnea monitor for a preterm infant sounds. The infant is asleep, the skin color is pink, and the heart rate is 130–135/min. The most appropriate initial nursing response is to: *(312)*
    1. contact the physician for orders.
    2. gently rub the infant's back.
    3. give oxygen with an Ambu bag.
    4. suction the infant with a bulb syringe.

12. A key nursing intervention to prevent retinopathy of prematurity is to: *(313; 315, Skill 13-1)*
    1. provide feedings as early as possible after birth.
    2. perform care to avoid moving the infant more than necessary.
    3. eliminate potential sources of infection from the environment.
    4. monitor the infant's blood oxygen levels.

13. Most problems of the postterm infant result from: *(321)*
    1. decreased functioning of the placenta.
    2. reduced blood clotting factors.
    3. increased susceptibility to infection.
    4. thicker subcutaneous fat deposits.

CASE STUDY

1. Kayla had a cesarean birth for reduction in amniotic fluid levels over 2 weeks. Michael was born at 35 weeks, 2 days (often abbreviated in practice as 35 2/7 weeks). The gestation makes Michael late preterm, although he weighs 3284 g (6 pounds, 10 ounces). At 6 hours of age, Michael became tachypneic with average respiratory rate of 70 per minute, but no grunting sounds. He is transferred to the special care nursery until the rapid respirations resolve in 1 1/2 days. Does this indicate a specific preterm problem? If so, which problem? See Chapter 14 for another possible problem.

THINKING CRITICALLY

1. A friend had her baby at 32 weeks gestation 6 months ago. She confides that she is afraid her baby is not normal because he does not do the same things her first baby (born at term) did at 6 months old. What can you tell your friend to reassure her?

APPLYING KNOWLEDGE

1. Observe newborns of different gestational ages in your clinical facility. Identify differences in these characteristics. Determine whether the mother's "due date" correlates with the physical characteristics you see. Do you note any differences if an infant is delivered by scheduled induction or cesarean?
   a. Head and body hair
   b. Body posture and muscle tone
   c. Stiffness of ear cartilage
   d. Amount of breast tissue
   e. Appearance of genitalia
   f. Number and depth of sole creases

2. Observe different methods of feeding preterm infants.
   a. What precautions are taken to ensure that the baby receives adequate nutrition without overload?
   b. Describe method(s) used in your facility to avoid bottle-feeding breast milk or formula if breastfeeding is planned as soon as possible for the baby.

3. If your facility does not routinely care for sick newborns, does it have arrangements with a larger hospital to transport these babies to a special care nursery? What is involved in transporting a sick baby? When do most newborns return to the original facility or are they usually discharged by the special care nursery in the larger hospital?

4. How does your facility foster parent-infant bonding when an infant is sick or preterm? Is kangaroo care used? Are facilities available for parents of the infant transported a long distance, such as Ronald McDonald houses?

5. Look up facility policies that relate to neonatal jaundice. Do specific definitions describe bilirubin levels and treatment for physiologic, pathologic, and breast milk jaundice?

The Newborn with a Perinatal Injury or Congenital Malformation

Answer Key: A complete answer key can be found on the Student Evolve website.

LEARNING ACTIVITIES

1. Match the terms in the left column with their definitions on the right (a–p).

_____ Cheiloplasty (331)

_____ Habilitation (329)

_____ Hydrocephalus (325)

_____ Hyperbilirubinemia (342)

_____ Kernicterus (342)

_____ Macrosomia (347, Fig. 14-17)

_____ Meningocele (328)

_____ Myelodysplasia (328)

_____ Meningomyelocele (328)

_____ Neonatal abstinence syndrome (346)

_____ Ortolani's sign (334)

_____ Pavlik harness (334, Fig. 14-10)

_____ Simian crease (339)

_____ Subluxation (333)

_____ Transillumination (325)

_____ Trisomy 21 (338)

a. Inspection of a cavity or organ by passing a light through its walls

b. Suggests developmental hip dysplasia

c. Teaching a skill to a child who is handicapped from birth

d. Maintains hip abduction in the treatment of developmental hip dysplasia

e. Single transverse line across the palm

f. Brain damage due to accumulation of bilirubin in the brain tissue

g. Large fetal or newborn body size

h. Surgical repair of a cleft lip

i. Partial displacement of the head of the femur from the acetabulum

j. Excess blood levels of bilirubin

k. Presence of one extra chromosome in a body cell

l. Group of malformations of the spinal cord

m. Accumulation of cerebrospinal fluid within the brain's ventricles

n. Form of spina bifida in which portions of the membranes and cerebrospinal fluid are contained in a cystic mass

o. Form of spina bifida that consists of protrusion of a saclike cyst containing meninges, spinal fluid, and a portion of the spinal cord with its nerves

p. Fetal exposure to maternal drugs that cause dependence

2. List five classes of congenital anomalies that may occur in the neonate. Give one or more examples of each. *(324; Box 14-1)*

   a. _____

   b. _____

   c. _____

   d. _____

   e. _____

3. List the two classifications of hydrocephalus and describe features of each. *(325)*

   a. _____

   _____

   b. _____

   _____

4. List two possible complications of shunts for treatment of hydrocephalus. *(326, Fig. 14-3)*

   a. _____

   b. _____

5. Why is it essential to frequently change position if an infant has an enlarged head due to hydrocephalus but has not yet had a shunt placed? *(327)*

   _____

   _____

6. List signs of the two primary complications that may occur after shunt placement for hydrocephalus. *(327-328)*

   a. Infection of the shunt: _____

   _____

   b. Increased intracranial pressure:_____

   _____

7. What is the current recommendation for all women related to prevention of neural tube defects such as meningomyelocele? *(328)*

   _____

   _____

8. Describe nursing observations and care for the newborn with spina bifida in each of the following areas. *(329-330)*

   a. Care of the sac before surgical repair:_____

   _____

    b.   Extremities: _____

_____

    c.   Head: _____

_____

    d.   Bowel and bladder function: _____

_____

    e.   Latex allergy: _____

_____

9.   What are the positioning options the nurse may use for a child with a myelocele or meningomyelocele before surgical repair? *(329)*

_____

_____

10. Describe postoperative nursing care for the child with a cleft lip and/or palate repair. *(331-332)*

    a.   Preventing injury to the operative site: _____

_____

    b.   Positioning: _____

_____

    c.   Prevention of infection: _____

_____

    d.   Emotional care: _____

_____

    e.   Pain relief: _____

_____

11. Describe three ways of treating clubfoot. *(332-333)*

    a.   _____

    b.   _____

    c.   _____

12. Describe nursing care of the child who has a cast on both legs. *(334-335)* _____

_____

_____

_____

_____

13. List four signs of developmental hip dysplasia in the infant. *(333-334)*

    a. _____

    b. _____

    c. _____

    d. _____

14. What procedure should the nurse use to turn a child in a body (spica) cast? *(334-335; 336, Skill 14-1; 336, Nursing Care Plan 14-1)*

    _____

    _____

    _____

    _____

15. a. Explain how and when the nurse will screen a newborn for phenylketonuria (PKU). Explain if the baby should be rechecked for PKU values and when. *(337)*

    _____

    _____

    _____

    b. An infant's initial PKU screening is positive. What confirmation test is done for positive results on a screening test? *(337)*

    _____

    _____

16. Describe the manifestations of the listed inborn errors of metabolism, how they are diagnosed, and their treatment. *(337-338)*

    a. Maple syrup urine disease: _____

    _____

    _____

    b. Galactosemia: _____

    _____

    _____

17. Describe physical and developmental characteristics that may be seen in a child with Down syndrome. *(338-340; Tables 14-1 and 14-2)*

    a. Facial features: _____

    _____

b. Hands and feet: _____

_____

c. Musculoskeletal characteristics: _____

_____

d. Internal abnormalities: _____

_____

e. Physical and intellectual development: _____

_____

18. Parents of children born with Down syndrome have special needs. Give examples of how the nurse could help parents meet these needs. *(340)*

a. Resistance to infection: _____

_____

b. Hypotonic muscles and loose joints:_____

_____

c. Constipation: _____

_____

d. Grieving: _____

_____

19. Describe occurrences in the pathophysiology of erythroblastosis fetalis. *(Boxes 14-2 and 14-3; Fig. 14-13; 340-341; Safety Alert)*

_____

_____

20. a. What drug can prevent development of erythroblastosis fetalis and who (mother or infant) should receive it? *(340; Box 14-2)*

_____

_____

b. List five circumstances in which the drug is indicated. *(341)*

i. _____

ii. _____

iii. _____

iv. _____

v. _____

21. Explain related nursing care in each of the following areas if an infant must receive phototherapy in an incubator rather than with a fiberoptic pad or blanket. *(342-344, Figs. 14-14, 14-15, and 14-16, Box 14-4, 345, Nursing Care Plan 14-2)*

    a. Eye protection: _____

    _____

    b. Protection of ovaries or testes: _____

    _____

    c. Potential dehydration: _____

    _____

22. Intracranial hemorrhage around the time of birth is usually caused by _____ or
    _____. *(345)*

23. List signs that should make the nurse suspect that a newborn has had an intracranial hemorrhage. *(345-346)*

    _____

    _____

    _____

    _____

24. What are two possible permanent effects of an intracranial hemorrhage? *(346)*

    a. _____

    b. _____

25. a. What causes the infants of some diabetic mothers to be larger than expected for their gestational age? *(347)*

    _____

    _____

    b. What are other possible outcomes for the infant when the woman has diabetes during pregnancy? *(347)*

    _____

    _____

    c. What blood test should the nurse expect to perform when a term infant is born to a diabetic mother? What is the normal level for a newborn? *(347)*

    _____

    _____

REVIEW QUESTIONS

1. A sign that should make the nurse suspect hydrocephalus in the newborn is: *(325)*
   1. inability to sleep between feedings.
   2. a patch of hair on the lower back.
   3. axillary temperature of 37.8° C (100° F).
   4. an enlarged fontanelle or cranial sutures.

2. Expected treatment for hydrocephalus is: *(326)*
   1. placement of a shunt.
   2. incision and draining.
   3. oral liquid diuretics.
   4. intravenous analgesics.

3. Vital sign changes when an infant has increased intracranial pressure include: *(327)*
   1. increased blood pressure and pulse, hyperventilation.
   2. decreased blood pressure, pulse, and respirations.
   3. decreased blood pressure and respirations, increased pulse.
   4. increased blood pressure, decreased pulse and respirations.

4. Before surgical repair, the usual position of a newborn with a meningomyelocele is: *(329)*
   1. side-lying with the head slightly below the level of the heart.
   2. prone, maintaining abduction with a pad between the legs.
   3. supine with the crib flat to stabilize blood pressure.
   4. supine with the legs widely abducted and thighs flexed.

5. Which nursing measure is appropriate for a 2-week-old infant who has a new cleft lip repair? *(331)*
   1. Position on the abdomen or side.
   2. Place in a car seat after each feeding.
   3. Provide a premature-sized pacifier.
   4. Limit visitors to immediate family.

6. A priority of postoperative nursing care for a 9-month-old infant who has cleft palate repair is: *(331)*
   1. referral to a parent support group.
   2. adequate nutrition.
   3. keeping an intravenous line open.
   4. continuous sedation.

7. Appropriate care related to a new plaster cast for correction of clubfoot in the newborn is to: *(333)*
   1. keep the infant snugly wrapped until the cast is dry to prevent hypothermia.
   2. sprinkle powder into the dry cast to reduce skin irritation at the edges of the cast.
   3. position with the feet lower than the level of the heart until the cast is dry.
   4. observe the toes for pallor, cyanosis, reduced capillary refill, or cold temperature.

8. When checking range of motion of an infant, what sign suggests developmental hip dysplasia? *(333)*
   1. Reduced thigh abduction
   2. Full abduction and adduction
   3. Equal gluteal creases in the back
   4. Limited flexion of one knee

9. A 2-week-old infant will be fitted with a Pavlik harness as treatment for developmental hip dysplasia. The mother asks the nurse about the harness and how it will help her baby. To reinforce the physician's explanation, the nurse should teach the mother that: *(334, Fig. 14-10)*
   1. keeping the hip bone within the hip socket helps the socket to become deeper.
   2. the infant cannot have surgery for the condition until he is at least 8 weeks old.
   3. the longer leg gradually becomes shorter to equalize the leg lengths before walking.
   4. time spent in a cast is reduced if the baby is treated with a harness for a few weeks.

10. The nurse should suspect intracranial hemorrhage in a newborn if: *(345-346)*
    1. the fontanelle is of normal size, but depressed.
    2. muscle tone has become poor since birth.
    3. the infant seems to be hungry much of the time.
    4. both pupils are small and react to light when checked.

11. The child with PKU must be on a diet that is: *(337, Safety Alert)*
    1. low in fatty acids to promote intellectual development.
    2. high in soluble fiber to reduce constipation.
    3. low in phenylalanine to limit buildup of the protein.
    4. fluid-restricted to reduce the wastes delivered to the kidneys.

12. Early identification of galactosemia is required to prevent: *(338)*
    1. depletion of specific amino acids.
    2. liver damage, cataracts, and mental retardation.
    3. protein deposits in the adrenal glands and kidneys.
    4. limitation of normal growth in height.

13. Appropriate nursing care for parents immediately after the birth of a baby who has characteristics typical of Down syndrome should include: *(340)*
    1. reassuring them that future babies are unlikely to have this problem.
    2. keeping the infant in the nursery until a definitive diagnosis is made.
    3. spending time with them so they can best verbalize their concerns.
    4. teaching them about lifelong nutritional care the baby will need.

14. Parent-infant bonding for an infant with a meningomyelocele prior to repair can be enhanced by: *(330)*
    1. encouraging the parents to talk to and touch the baby.
    2. having the parents change the baby's diaper.
    3. encouraging the parents to hold the baby near their skin.
    4. helping a parent give the baby an admission bath.

15. The mother of a 2-week-old infant who is going to have a cleft lip repair asks if she will be able to hold her baby after surgery. The nurse should reply: *(331)*
    1. "The baby can be held when she no longer needs the restraints."
    2. "The baby cannot be held but you can talk to her and stroke her."
    3. "Holding your baby helps keep her content."
    4. "You should hold your baby only during feedings."

16. An Rh-negative woman who gives birth to an Rh-positive infant should receive $Rh_o(D)$ immune globulin (RhoGAM) no later than _____ hours after birth. *(341; Nursing Tip)*
    1. 4–8
    2. 16
    3. 24–36
    4. 72

17. Expected advice for the woman with PKU who is considering pregnancy is to eat a daily diet that: *(337)*
    1. contains additional high-fiber foods.
    2. contains adequate dairy products.
    3. provides added amounts of leucine.
    4. has low quantities of phenylalanine.

18. The infant with Down syndrome is at increased risk for developing: *(339)*
    1. urinary tract infections.
    2. respiratory infections.
    3. kidney infections.
    4. meningitis.

19. What complication is more likely for an infant of a diabetic mother within the first few hours after birth? *(347; see also Chapter 5)*
    1. Intracranial hemorrhage
    2. Hyperactive reflexes
    3. Excessive urination
    4. Low blood glucose levels

20. Why might an infant of a diabetic mother be small for gestational age (SGA)? *(347)*
    1. The placenta did not receive adequate perfusion during pregnancy.
    2. The fetus had episodes of hypoglycemia when the mother took insulin.
    3. The fetal pancreas does not make insulin if the mother takes insulin.
    4. The mother's diabetes causes small areas of bleeding in the placenta.

21. Meconium aspiration syndrome may be prevented by: *(346)*
    1. stimulating the infant to breathe as soon as delivery is complete.
    2. reducing meconium in amniotic fluid before birth by amnioinfusion.
    3. intubating the infant immediately after birth for ventilation.
    4. promoting adequate infant oxygenation with an apnea monitor.

CASE STUDIES

1. A term newborn who has a meningomyelocele has paralysis of the legs and is dribbling urine and stool. Surgical closure of the spinal defect has not yet been done.
   a. Identify four nursing concerns for the nurse caring for the baby.
   b. Neonatal physicians and pediatric neurosurgeons have talked with parents about probable permanent effects that will remain after surgery. How can the nurse reinforce needed newborn care related to the dribbling of urine and oozing of stool and effects on skin care? Describe possible future techniques to help control of these functions.
   c. How should the nurse involve the parents in the infant's care in the newborn nursery, both preoperatively and postoperatively?
   d. What related problems should the nurse observe for in this infant? What signs should make the nurse suspect that the problems have developed?

2. Breanna, 4 months old, is brought to the hospital by her mother because she had a seizure this morning. The admission physical exam shows an irritable, thin, lethargic child who the mother says has been vomiting the small amount of formula she would eat. Her height and weight measurements are below normal and her head circumference is slightly larger than normal. Breanna has not had any health care since her birth in a distant city. The admitting diagnosis is suspected hydrocephalus.
   a. Is Breanna exhibiting any signs of increased intracranial pressure? List observations that would support your conclusion.
   b. List diagnostic tests that may be done to confirm this diagnosis.
   c. What nursing measures should the nurse take to promote skin integrity?
   d. How should the nurse position Breanna during and after feedings?

APPLYING KNOWLEDGE

1. If you have a pediatric patient with Down syndrome (trisomy 21), compare the development of gross and fine motor abilities of the child with those of a child of the same approximate age who does not have Down syndrome. Has the child with Down syndrome had any of the associated problems such as respiratory infections, ear infections, or heart defects?

2. While in the clinical area, care for a child or adult who has Down syndrome. If you have a friend or family member with Down syndrome, consider telling your classmates what you have learned over time.

3. Observe the repair of a cleft lip or cleft palate. If unable to observe an existing cleft or its repair, observe the results of a repair from a future patient if possible.

4. Care for an infant receiving phototherapy with a fiberoptic pad or blanket. What is the most likely cause for the hyperbilirubinemia in this child? Are term infants discharged from your facility for home phototherapy? What procedures are followed for starting and follow-up of home phototherapy? Is exposure to natural light utilized to reduce bilirubin levels?

5. Give $Rh_O(D)$ immune globulin (RhoGAM) under instructor supervision. Why is this patient having the medication at this time? If you have clinical or have worked in an obstetrics and gynecology clinic, ask which women are likely to receive RhoGAM and when during their pregnancy.

6. What should you teach a parent, teen, or adult about caring for a cast, such as one for an arm fracture? If you now work in an emergency department (not as a nurse but as a medical assistant or tech), what type of casts have you seen applied?

An Overview of Growth, Development, and Nutrition

LEARNING ACTIVITIES

1. Match the terms in the left column with their definitions on the right (a–f).

_____ Cephalocaudal *(353, Fig. 15-1)*	a. Progressive increase in physical size
_____ Development *(352, Box 15-2 and Box 15-3, Fig. 15-1)*	b. Progressive increase in body function
	c. Total way a person grows and develops, dictated by inheritance
_____ Growth *(352, Box 15-2 and Box 15-3, Fig. 15-1)*	d. Head-to-toe developmental pattern
_____ Maturation *(352, Box 15-3, Fig. 15-1)*	e. Central-to-peripheral developmental pattern
_____ Parallel play *(384, Table 15-10)*	f. Activity alongside another child or children
_____ Proximodistal *(353, Box 15-3, Fig. 15-1)*	

2. True or false?

   a. Children grow at a steady rate and in an orderly process. *(352, Fig. 15-1)* _____

   b. Development proceeds from simple to complex. *(350, Box 15-1)* _____

3. State the age range for each of the following stages of development. Use markers such as events, days, weeks, months, or years that are appropriate for the stage. *(352)*

   a. Fetus: _____

   b. Newborn: _____

   c. Infant: _____

   d. Toddler: _____

   e. Preschool child: _____

   f. School-age child: _____

   g. Adolescent: _____

4. Give a specific example of each type of developmental pattern. *(353, Figure 15-1)*

   a. Cephalocaudal:_____

   b. Proximodistal: _____

5. What are the two most rapid periods of growth after birth? *(353)*

    a. _____

    b. _____

6. Birth weight usually _____ by 6 months of age and _____ by 1 year. *(353)*

7. How does the percentage of body fluid change as the infant matures to adulthood? Why is it important for the nurse to know this? *(353)*

    _____

    _____

    _____

8. Why would a burn chart for calculating percentage of injured body surface area for an adult be inappropriate for a child with burns? *(352, Figure 15-2)*

    _____

    _____

    _____

9. Why are ear infections more common in young children? *(353)* _____

    _____

    _____

    _____

10. What factors contribute to the development of physiologic anemia in a 3-month-old infant? *(354)*

    _____

    _____

11. Infants are susceptible to dehydration because _____
    _____. *(353, 355)*

12. The Denver II assesses the _____ status of children from birth to 6 years of age in the following four categories: *(356)*

    a. _____

    b. _____

    c. _____

    d. _____

13. True or false?

    a. The Denver II is an intelligence test. *(356)* _____

    b. A low score on the Denver II indicates that a child has a developmental delay. *(356)* _____

    c. A dysfunctional family implies its members are not loving and caring. *(359)* _____

14. List five factors that can influence a child's growth and development. *(356)*

    a. _____

    b. _____

    c. _____

    d. _____

    e. _____

15. How can physical illness affect a child's growth and development? *(356)* _____

    _____

16. List the components of the family Apgar. *(360)*

    A _____

    P _____

    G _____

    A _____

    R _____

17. Define *systems theory*. *(360)* _____

    _____

    _____

    _____

18. Match the following behaviors with the correct stages of Piaget's theory of cognitive development (a–d). *(368, Table 15-3)*

    _____ Sensorimotor

    _____ Preoperational

    _____ Concrete operations

    _____ Formal operations

    a. Progresses from reflexes to intentional interaction with the environment
    b. Develops ability for hypothetical and abstract thought
    c. Views the world egocentrically
    d. Reasoning becomes logical; understands cause and effect

19. Describe the moral development of a 5-year-old child. *(368, Table 15-3)* _____

    _____

    _____

    _____

20. How can parents' knowledge of growth and development help prevent accidents in children? *(352)*

_____

_____

_____

_____

21. Why might a child who eats a vegetarian diet be anemic? *(357, Fig. 15-7, Nutrition Considerations box; 371)*

_____

_____

_____

_____

22. What is the food of choice for the first 6 months to 1 year of life? *(373)*_____

_____

23. Why are restrictive diets not recommended for infants and young children? *(373)* _____

_____

24. The first solid food introduced to infants is usually _____ _____. *(375; 377, Fig. 15-9)*

25. Solid foods are introduced into the infant's diet at what age? *(377)*_____

26. What is the earliest age that a child should begin whole milk? *(377, Nursing Tip)*_____

27. One guideline for determining the appropriate amount of food to feed to children is _____ tablespoon(s) of food for each year of age. *(380)*

28. Primary dentition is completed by _____ years. *(380; 381, Figure 15-12)*

29. The first primary teeth erupt at _____ months. *(381, Fig. 15-12)*

30. True or false?

    a. Carbohydrate consumption is the most important dietary consideration for dental health. *(381)*
        _____

    b. The child should be encouraged to brush his or her teeth after eating sticky foods. *(381)* _____

    c. The American Academy of Pediatric Dentistry recommends that children have their first dental visit by 1 year of age. *(380)* _____

31. a. What are the causes of bottle-mouth caries? *(382, Fig. 15-14)* _____

        _____

        _____

    b. What is the prevention measure for them? *(382)* _____

        _____

32. Administration of _____ after age _____ is important to prevent dental caries. *(381)*

33. What is the first-aid measure for traumatic loss of a permanent tooth? *(383)* _____

_____

_____

_____

34. What is the chief difference between the play of several toddlers (ages 1–2 years) and play of several preschoolers (ages 3–5 years)? *(384, Table 15-10)*

_____

_____

_____

REVIEW QUESTIONS

1. A child must be able to sit before he can walk. This is an example of which directional pattern of development? *(353)*
   1. Cephalocaudal
   2. Proportional
   3. Proximodistal
   4. Linear

2. One of the most accurate indicators of biologic age is: *(355)*
   1. height.
   2. weight.
   3. bone growth.
   4. teeth eruption.

3. The nurse instructs the parent of an infant that dental caries are prevented through the administration of oral: *(376, Table 15-8)*
   1. iodine.
   2. fluoride.
   3. sodium.
   4. iron.

4. Most children are able to feed themselves using a spoon by age: *(351, Box 15-1)*
   1. 1 year.
   2. 2 years.
   3. 3 years.
   4. 4 years.

5. The theorist known for his work on moral development is: *(367)*
   1. Freud.
   2. Kohlberg.
   3. Erikson.
   4. Piaget.

6. A current comic strip depicts a family in which parents, children, and the children's grandfather live together. This is an example of a(n): *(359)*
   1. nuclear family.
   2. biologic family.
   3. extended family.
   4. blended family.

7. Blood cholesterol below which level is considered acceptable in children older than 2 years and adolescents? *(375, Box 5-4)*
   1. <170 mg/dL
   2. <180 mg/dL
   3. <200 mg/dL
   4. <220 mg/dL

8. The nurse understands that primary dentition is usually completed by age: *(380)*
   1. 18 months.
   2. 2½ years.
   3. 4 years
   4. 6 years.

9. An infant weighed 7 pounds, 11 ounces (3487 g) at birth. What would the nurse expect this infant to weigh at 12 months of age? *(353)*
   1. 15 pounds (6.8 kg)
   2. 20 pounds (9 kg)
   3. 23 pounds (10.4 kg)
   4. 25 pounds (11.2 kg)

10. Which statement would have the most positive outcome when the nurse is counseling adolescents on nutrition? *(379)*
    1. "If you don't eat properly now, you may have heart trouble when you get older."
    2. "You will get run down and sick if you don't eat properly."
    3. "Shiny hair and good muscles are linked to good nutrition."
    4. "If you eat nutritiously, you won't have acne."

11. Young children are playing with action figures in the hospital playroom. Closer observation reveals they are playing alongside one another, rather than interacting with each other. The nurse is observing: *(384; Table 15-10)*
    1. solitary play.
    2. parallel play.
    3. cooperative play.
    4. creative play.

12. The nurse determines a parent needs additional teaching about nutrition when the parent states: *(376, Table 15-8; 382)*
    1. "My 2-year-old child uses a spoon to feed himself."
    2. "I feed my 8-month-old infant iron-fortified cereal."
    3. "My 1-year-old infant falls asleep with a bottle of formula."
    4. "I give my 3-year-old 3 tablespoons of vegetables."

13. The nurse would teach a parent to introduce solid foods to an infant at what age? *(376, Table 15-8; 377, Fig. 15-9)*
    1. 3 months
    2. 6 months
    3. 8 months
    4. 10 months

14. What is the best nursing response to a parent who asks when her 3-month-old infant can switch from iron-fortified formula to milk? *(377, Nursing Tip)*
    1. "Switch to milk when you introduce solid foods."
    2. "The baby can have milk when she can drink from a cup."
    3. "Milk can be given at 6 months of age."
    4. "Infants can drink milk after their first birthday."

15. A 4-year-old child had a low score on the Denver II. The nurse understands that this finding indicates: *(356)*
    1. there is a need for further evaluation.
    2. the child has a cognitive impairment.
    3. there is a problem with the child's speech.
    4. the child has a developmental delay.

16. Which statement made by a parent indicates an understanding about a child's dental health? *(383)*
    1. "I give my son a new toothbrush every year on his birthday."
    2. "I rinse the toothbrush bristles in hot water after my son brushes."
    3. "My 1-year-old brushes his teeth all by himself every day."
    4. "I replaced the toothbrush after my son had a sore throat."

17. The nurse is assessing the nutritional status of a 6-year-old child. Which finding suggests the child is well-nourished? *(379)*
    1. Protuberant abdomen
    2. Pale oral mucous membranes
    3. Alert and energetic
    4. Coarse, thin hair

18. The nurse should teach the mother of a 19-month-old which action(s) to recommend best oral care? Select all that apply. *(381; 382, Health Promotion)*
    1. "If fussy at bedtime, give the baby about 1/2 cup of clear juice in a bottle."
    2. "Brush your baby's teeth before bedtime each night."
    3. "Fluoride is beneficial to the teeth of a child at this age."
    4. "Children will have permanent teeth to replace any 'baby teeth' they lose."
    5. "Water in a bottle is safe for teeth at any time."
    6. "Add toothbrushes for your family to a dishwasher load once a week for thorough cleaning."

CASE STUDY

1. You are assigned to observe and interact with a group of 6 children at a day care center for employees at the hospital where you are assigned to clinical. Children in this group are 3 and 4 years old.
   a. Describe the play activities that you would expect among this group.
   b. Describe appropriate snacks for the group and when you think is a good time to serve the snacks during their day at the center.
   c. Is a nap reasonable? If so, how did the children handle naptime?
   d. Tour the day care facility where assigned and see variations in toys, furnishings and equipment, ratio of children to caregivers in specific rooms, and other items of interest.

THINKING CRITICALLY

1. Observe a child in the clinical area. Based on the assessment, determine which of Erikson's stages of development the child is attempting to accomplish. Give at least three examples of observed behavior that support your choice. Your clinical teacher may also assign you or a small group to a child for evaluation. This may be a well child in day care rather than a patient.

2. Using the information provided in Table 15-6 in the textbook and the Food Guide Pyramid (Figure 15-6), develop a meal plan for a 9-year-old child using foods unique to that child's ethnic background.

APPLYING KNOWLEDGE

1. a. Plot the height and weight of the following children on the growth chart (Figure 15-3 in the textbook). What are the age, height or length, and weight of the most recent pediatric patient that you cared for in clinical?

Age	Height	Weight
2 years (boy)	33 in. (83.8 cm)	26 lbs. (11.79 kg)
4 years (girl)	38 in. (96.5 cm)	43 lbs. (19.5 kg)
8 years (boy)	52 in. (132 cm)	60 lbs. (27.2 kg)
12 years (girl)	58 in. (147 cm)	65 lbs. (29.5 kg)

   b. What percentile does each of the above children fall into?
   c. Which child would need further evaluation of his or her growth?
   d. Do you have a height/length and the weight for a child whom you have cared for recently, including your own child? Make inch to centimeter and pound/ounce to gram/kilogram conversions as appropriate for the size of this child.

2. Plan a menu for a 4-year-old hospitalized child on a general diet. Include in your plan serving size and how the food is best served.

3. Perform a developmental assessment using the Denver II. Discuss your experience with your classmates.

The Infant

Answer Key: A complete answer key can be found on the Student Evolve website.

LEARNING ACTIVITIES

1. Match the terms in the left column with their definitions on the right (a–h).

   _____ Colic *(395; 391, Box 16-1)*
   _____ Creep *(389, Fig. 16-3; 393, Box 16-1)*
   _____ Extrusion reflex *(397)*
   _____ Grasp reflex *(387)*
   _____ Object permanence *(404, Table 16-4)*
   _____ Parachute reflex *(387)*
   _____ Pincer grasp *(387)*
   _____ Prehension *(387)*

   a. Closure of the hand when the palm is touched or stroked
   b. Thrusting tongue movements that automatically push food out of the mouth
   c. Extension of both arms when thrust downward in the prone position
   d. Ability to grasp objects between all fingers of one hand and the opposing thumb of the same hand
   e. Self-propelled forward movement carrying trunk above and parallel to floor
   f. Accurate and coordinated opposition of index finger and thumb of same hand
   g. Infant can remember that an object exists even if it is out of sight
   h. Unexplained episodes of crying and irritability in an otherwise healthy infant

2. How does sucking benefit a young infant? *(387)*

   a. _____

   b. _____

3. How can the nurse help meet the infant's sucking needs during the following? *(387, Fig. 16-2)*

   a. Oral feedings: _____

   _____

   _____

   b. Intravenous fluid therapy: _____

   _____

   _____

4. a. The primary goal for normal personality development during infancy is to acquire a sense of
_____. *(387)*

   b. What can the nurse teach parents about meeting this need of their infant? *(387)* _____

   _____

   _____

5. Appropriate sensory stimulation is needed to promote what type of infant development? *(388)*

   a. _____

   b. _____

6. At how many months of age are the following events in an infant's growth and development likely to occur? *(390, Box 16-1)*
   a. Briefly holds head erect and in the midline of body _____
   b. Feeds self finger foods _____
   c. Should have first DTP (diphtheria, tetanus, pertussis) immunization _____
   d. Two lower central incisors; begins to crawl; transfers objects from one hand to the other _____
   e. Birth weight tripled; may walk _____
   f. Sits alone; pincer grasp _____
   g. Walks holding furniture; deliberately throws objects on floor _____
   h. Turns from back to side _____
   i. Can place a toy in small container _____
   j. "Jumps" when in lap of caregiver _____

7. a. Why should most infants not be placed in the prone position for sleep? *(395; Safety Alert, 396)* _____

   _____

   _____

   b. Give examples of measures to reduce an infant's risk of suffocation. *(396, Safety Alert)* _____

   _____

   _____

8. What are three points that the nurse should emphasize to parents to promote childhood immunization? *(397)*

   a. _____

   b. _____

   c. _____

9. What guidance can the nurse give new parents who are concerned about whether their baby is receiving an adequate diet of breast milk or formula? *(397)*

   a. _____

   b. _____

   c. _____

10. List four assessments that the health care provider may use to gauge the adequacy of an infant's nutrition. *(397)*

    a. _____

    b. _____

    c. _____

    d. _____

11. List health benefits of breastfeeding an infant. *(397-398)*

    a. _____

    b. _____

    c. _____

    d. _____

12. What food should be avoided until the child is 1 year old? Why should this food be avoided? Explain how you would avoid the food. *(401, Health Promotion, Safety Alert)*

    _____

    _____

    _____

13. a. What is the current recommendation about when solid foods may be introduced to the infant's diet? *(401)*

    _____

    _____

    b. Why is this a good age to begin introducing solid foods? *(401)* _____

    _____

    _____

14. a. What is the first solid food usually introduced to the infant? *(401)* _____

    _____

    b. Why is this food good as an introductory solid food? *(401)* _____

    _____

15. How should parents introduce new solid foods so that an infant's tolerance or intolerance of the food can be identified? *(401)*

    _____

    _____

16. List six foods that are usually avoided until the baby is 1 year old. Why is addition of these foods often delayed? *(401)*

    a. _____

    b. _____

    c. _____

    d. _____

    e. _____

    f. _____

17. The United States population is becoming more obese, causing multiple health problems. Is feeding an infant a low-fat diet one answer to the problem? Give a reason for your answer. *(402)*

    _____

    _____

REVIEW QUESTIONS

1. The priority need in personality development during the first year is to acquire: *(387)*
   1. fear when meeting strangers.
   2. mastering self-feeding.
   3. trust in the primary caregivers.
   4. regular sleeping, waking, and feeding.

2. The primary use of growth and development guidelines is to: *(396)*
   1. help parents anticipate their child's changing needs.
   2. compare children of similar ages with each other.
   3. predict general intelligence and school performance.
   4. identify the child who may be mentally retarded.

3. Which developmental milestone is appropriate for each child's age in the selection below? *(390-393, Box 16-1)*
   1. Passes a toy from one hand to the other at 3 months.
   2. Uses the root reflex to seek the nipple at 5 months.
   3. Sits steadily alone with a straight back at 6 months.
   4. Pulls self to standing position at 10 months.

4. The mother of a 2-month-old is bringing her to the office for a routine checkup and immunizations. She says the baby cries quite a bit but she just lets her cry so she won't become "spoiled." As a nurse, the best response is to: *(386; Nursing Care Plan 16-1)*
   1. tell the mother she should also lower the lights and play soft music or other "white noise."
   2. explain that babies this young cannot be spoiled, then give her some ideas to help soothe the baby and instill trust.
   3. encourage the mother to continue helping her baby become more independent.
   4. reassure the mother that she has an irritable baby, but that this phase will not continue for long.

5. The best position for a newborn to sleep is: *(396)*
   1. on the abdomen.
   2. in an infant seat.
   3. with the caregiver.
   4. supine or side-lying.

6. If a parent wants to microwave formula before feeding, the nurse should: *(399, 401)*
   1. explain that microwaving heats formula unevenly and can cause severe burns.
   2. tell the parent that cold formula preserves the nutrients better than heating it.
   3. advise the parent to wait until the infant takes at least 8 ounces of formula at each feeding.
   4. tell the parent that formula heats less evenly than breast milk and to mix and test very carefully.

7. The primary focus of regular infant health care is to: *(396)*
   1. prevent disease.
   2. accelerate development.
   3. delay onset of allergies.
   4. assess growth rate.

8. A mother wants to know if she can keep leftover baby food in a jar. Choose the best nursing response. *(402)*
   1. "If you heard a definite 'pop' when opening the jar, refrigerating leftovers is safe."
   2. "Refrigerate the leftover food within 2 hours after it is opened."
   3. "When the baby has eaten all she wants from the jar, promptly refrigerate the remainder."
   4. "Remove the amount of food you think the baby will eat from the jar and refrigerate the rest."

9. A formula often prescribed for the infant with galactosemia is based on: *(399)*
   1. goat's milk.
   2. soy.
   3. rice.
   4. artificial protein.

10. A nurse counsels a mother who is starting her baby on solid foods that she should wait _____ days before introducing the next food. *(401)*
    1. 1–2
    2. 2–3
    3. 4–7
    4. 7–14

11. Social development that is common for the 2-month-old infant is: *(390, Box 16-1)*
    1. responsive smiling.
    2. laughing aloud.
    3. recognizing his/her own name.
    4. anxiety around strangers.

12. When bringing her 9-month-old baby in for a checkup, a new mother asks if she can feed the baby puréed fish since this is a low-fat food that is a staple in the family's diet. The best response of the nurse is: *(401)*
    1. "It is never too early to begin a heart-healthy diet."
    2. "Fish protein is one of the best quality proteins available."
    3. "You can try, but many infants dislike the taste of fish."
    4. "Fish is more likely than other meats to cause allergies."

13. The parents should make safety preparations prior to the time their infant crawls, usually about age: *(392, Box 16-1)*
    1. 4 months.
    2. 7 months.
    3. 10 months.
    4. 12 months.

14. Which is the most important teaching about use of the microwave for heating infant food? *(399, 401)*
    1. Use less time than would be needed for larger pieces of food.
    2. Rotate the food two or more times while warming it.
    3. Avoid heating foods that are higher in fat, such as meat.
    4. Test the temperature of any warmed food on the inner wrist.

15. A fruit that should be delayed until after the infant's first birthday is: *(401)*
    1. strawberries.
    2. applesauce.
    3. apricots.
    4. pears.

16. Considering safety when choosing toys for a 5-month-old, one should assume that all of them will go into the baby's: *(387)*
    1. tub.
    2. food.
    3. mouth.
    4. bed.

17. Minor head lag when pulling a 1-month-old infant to the sitting position: *(390, Box 16-1)*
    1. is an expected finding.
    2. demonstrates prematurity.
    3. identifies poor nutrition.
    4. suggests developmental delay.

18. A mother is concerned because her 1-year-old, who was 7 pounds (3178 g) at birth is "getting fat." The baby now weighs 21 pounds and all developmental milestones have been reached at appropriate ages. What should the nurse tell the mother about her baby's weight? *(394, Box 16-1)*
    1. The weight at 12 months is about twice the birth weight.
    2. The baby's weight gain is what is expected at this age.
    3. A low-fat diet helps avoid being overweight later in life.
    4. Infants normally weigh about 25 pounds by 1 year.

19. The nurse can reassure parents that their infant's colic will probably not last beyond the age of: *(390, Box 16-1)*
    1. 1 month.
    2. 3 months.
    3. 6 months.
    4. 9 months.

20. The baby can usually be offered finger foods such as toast or Zwieback crackers beginning at about age: *(392, Box 16-1)*
    1. 3 months.
    2. 5 months.
    3. 7 months.
    4. 9 months.

21. A good initial method to deal with a 9-month-old infant who is attracted to a dangerous situation is to: *(387; 393, Box 16-1)*
    1. shout a quick, loud "no."
    2. take his favorite toys away.
    3. spank him with one light blow.
    4. distract him from the situation.

CASE STUDIES

1. You are answering questions from the parents of Riley, a healthy newborn, in each of the following areas. Formulate appropriate parent teaching.
   a. Immunizations (first year) (In addition to Box 16-1, see the American Academy of Pediatrics at www.aap.org or the Centers for Disease Control at www.cdc.gov for the latest updates about immunization recommendations.)
   b. Sleeping all night (Describe how you, a friend, or a family member soothed a baby back to sleep. Do you think the method worked well? What are some alternatives that you might suggest?)
   c. Colic

2. Isaiah, a 6-month-old, is visiting the clinic for his immunizations and checkup. His parents will begin feeding solid foods now. What should you teach his parents in each of the following areas?
   a. Order of introducing solid foods
   b. Foods to avoid and how long to avoid them
   c. Avoiding infections acquired from foods

THINKING CRITICALLY

1. A mother is concerned because her 4-month-old baby does not seem to be developing as quickly as her sister's baby, who is about the same age. What should the nurse tell this mother about infant development?

APPLYING KNOWLEDGE

1. Determine the most common infant formulas recommended by physicians or pediatric nurse-practitioners in your clinical facility.
   a. What special infant formulas are readily available in the newborn nursery or the pediatric unit and when are these prescribed?
   b. Check a grocery, drug, or discount store to compare prices for each formula.

2. Ask a mother who has breastfed a previous child about her experience.
   a. Did she pump breast milk and was the milk fed to the baby by bottle?
   b. How old was the child when he or she stopped nursing?
   c. If the woman you talk with has just given birth to her second or later baby, how does she feel her experience of breastfeeding an older child will affect nursing her newest infant?

3. When caring for an infant in the pediatric unit, talk with parents about their baby's personality.
   a. Is their infant irritable, crying with handling or other stimulation, or calm when handled or meeting new people?
   b. How does the infant's behavior affect the parents or other family members?
   c. What, if any, different infant behavior do they notice while the baby is in the pediatric unit?

4. Ask several parents who had a colicky infant about their care.
   a. How long did the infant have colic? How did it affect the family?
   b. Was this their first or a later infant?
   c. Did you or a classmate have an experience with colic in your child or a family member's child? What actions helped?

The Toddler

Answer Key: A complete answer key can be found on the Student Evolve website.

LEARNING ACTIVITIES

1. Match the terms in the left column with their definitions on the right (a–g).

   _____ Autonomy *(406)*
   _____ Cooperative play *(418)*
   _____ Egocentric *(418)*
   _____ Negativism *(406)*
   _____ Parallel play *(418)*
   _____ Ritualism *(406)*
   _____ Separation anxiety *(408)*

   a. Independent play in company of other children
   b. Playing with other children
   c. Consistent, recurring pattern of behavior
   d. Independent functioning
   e. Thinking in reference to oneself
   f. Frequent reaction of "no"
   g. Protest, despair, and detachment related to temporary absence of caregiver

2. What age is the toddler is expected to achieve each developmental milestone? *(407, Table 17-1)*

   a. Can undress self, throws ball: _____

   b. All deciduous teeth are erupted; complete bowel and bladder control: _____

   c. Imitates adults' activities, holds spoon: _____

3. According to Erikson, the major developmental task for the toddler is to acquire _____ and overcome _____ and _____. *(406)*

4. What are the expected average vital signs for a 2-year-old? *(408)*

   a. Pulse: _____ to _____ bpm

   b. Respirations: _____ breaths/minute

   c. Blood pressure: _____ mm Hg

5. Describe each of these normal developmental processes. How can danger to a child occur related to expected development? Describe observations you have made of children related to each. *(406, 408)*

   a. Separation anxiety: _____

   _____

   _____

b. Object permanence: _____

_____

_____

6. What is a good guideline to teach parents about using "time out" with children? *(410)* _____

_____

7. List two self-consoling behaviors that toddlers exhibit. *(410)*

a. _____

b. _____

8. How should an adult talk to a toddler? Why? *(410)* _____

_____

9. List four indications of readiness for toilet training (in any order). *(411, Table 17-4; 412)*

a. _____

b. _____

c. _____

d. _____

10. Bladder training is more likely to succeed if the toddler stays dry for about _____ hours. *(412)*

11. Why is it important to teach the toddler generally recognized words to signal a need to use the bathroom? *(412)*

_____

_____

_____

_____

12. a. What deficiency is more likely to occur if a toddler has excessive milk and too few solid foods? *(413)*

_____

b. This can result in what condition? *(413)* _____

_____

13. Describe two characteristics of the toddler's eating habits.

a. Appetite: *(413)* _____

b. Food preferences: *(413)* _____

14. What guideline can the nurse give parents about serving size of solid foods? *(413)* _____

_____

15. List interventions that can assist parents with the toddler who resists bedtime. *(411, Table 17-4)*

a. _____

b. _____

c. _____

d. _____

e. _____

f. _____

16. _____ are the leading cause of childhood death. *(414)*

17. List two methods that are mandated by law to prevent injuries in children. *(417, Health Promotion box)*

a. _____

b. _____

REVIEW QUESTIONS

1. A first-time mother is concerned because she believes her 18-month-old son is not growing properly. Assessment indicates that the little boy's height and weight are average for his age. How can the nurse best advise her? *(406)*
   1. "He will soon resume the rapid growth of the first year."
   2. "It is normal for a child's growth to slow down after the first year."
   3. "Toddlers grow at inconsistent rates, much like adolescents."
   4. "The physician will do testing if your son's growth remains slow."

2. When helping a toddler choose clothing for the day, the best approach is to: *(406)*
   1. ask him what he wants to wear.
   2. ask which of two appropriate outfits he prefers.
   3. select the best outfit for the weather.
   4. remove all inappropriate clothing from his closet.

3. The position that best facilitates adult-child conversation is: *(410)*
   1. at the child's eye level.
   2. above the child's eye level.
   3. standing while the child sits.
   4. both seated at a small table.

4. When teaching parents of the toddler about eating, the nurse should stress that the toddler: *(413)*
   1. prefers a variety of foods mixed on the plate.
   2. must usually be coaxed to eat adequately.
   3. eats one food for a while, then rejects it.
   4. usually enjoys regular addition of new foods.

5. The mother of a 2-year-old asks the nurse whether she should begin toilet training now. The most appropriate nursing response is: *(412)*
   1. "Waiting about 6 months will improve the child's success with training."
   2. "Does your child ever wake up dry in the morning?"
   3. "Is it important to you and your family that the child be trained now?"
   4. "All children should be trained by age 2½, so you've got a while."

6. Automobile child restraint devices should be used when the child: *(417; Health Promotion)*
   1. begins sitting in the rear seat.
   2. crawls about in the car.
   3. becomes physically active.
   4. travels anywhere in the car.

7. Select the toy that is most likely to injure a toddler. *(415, Health Promotion)*
   1. Balloon
   2. Blocks
   3. Sand box
   4. Pull toy

8. Which is the best description of a 2-year-old's speech and language ability? *(408)*
   1. Naming objects precedes the ability to describe what they do.
   2. Some words such as swearing are used because they shock adults.
   3. Talking to the child delays clear speech by limiting time to practice.
   4. The child understands more than he or she is able to verbalize.

9. Choose the best description of physical changes during the toddler years. *(406-407)*
   1. Head growth slows and chest growth continues.
   2. Muscle size and strength remain steady.
   3. Body temperature regulation is erratic.
   4. Risk for infections is greater than during infancy.

10. The nurse can help reduce accidental injuries to toddlers by: *(414)*
    1. providing toys that help accelerate motor development.
    2. teaching parents about expected behavioral changes.
    3. providing written information about common childhood hazards.
    4. using restraints whenever the child is uncooperative.

11. Select the assessment that should make a parent or health care provider suspect a communication disorder. *(409, Table 17-3)*
    1. An 18-month-old child does not respond when his name is called.
    2. A 15-month-old child can point to one picture when the parent calls its name.
    3. A 3-year-old child can use plurals and pronouns correctly.
    4. A 16-month-old child cannot use two-word phrases when appropriate.

12. When assessing a 2-year-old child hospitalized for minor day surgery, the nurse should expect that the pulse rate will be about _____ bpm. *(408)*
    1. 60–80
    2. 70–110
    3. 125–135
    4. 120–140

13. When buying shoes for their toddler, parents should choose those that provide: *(412)*
    1. a firm, straight sole to facilitate walking.
    2. a strong arch to prevent "fallen" arches.
    3. protection from objects that might injure the feet.
    4. adequate movement of the heel within the shoe.

14. Choose the recommendation that best helps promote safety for the toddler. *(416, Health Promotion)*
    1. Keep medicines on a shelf rather than on the countertop.
    2. Provide stickers for each phone with the poison control center number.
    3. Advise parents to have a cell phone with them when driving.
    4. Use a hair dryer to dry the child's hair after shampooing to avoid colds.

15. A mother asks you what she should do about her 2-year-old child's temper tantrums. The best response is: *(411, Table 17-4)*
    1. "He is trying to tell you that he needs more attention from you and other important adults."
    2. "If you let him get away with temper tantrums now, he will have more problems later."
    3. "Have you tried rewarding his good behavior?"
    4. "Try putting him in his room for about 30 minutes."

CASE STUDY

1. Jacob is a 2-year-old whose mother is frustrated because of his temper tantrums when he is disciplined.
    a. What can you teach Jacob's mother about discipline at his age?
    b. How can knowledge of normal growth and development be used to teach his mother about setting limits?

THINKING CRITICALLY

1. A 14-month-old toddler has been pulling up and moving around furniture such as the coffee table but is not yet walking alone more than a few steps. He actively crawls around the home, often following his parents.
    a. List appropriate reminder precautions to teach parents about burns in the home that are appropriate for a toddler and often an older child or adult.
    b. Look in your text and online for information about childproofing the bathroom.
        i. List methods to teach parents about baby-proofing their bathroom with their child at the toddler age.
        ii. Why is this parent teaching especially important for toddlers? Think of what the toddler's parents should check at a home with no young children.
        iii. List all websites that you use for parent teaching information.
    c. What did you learn about toddler safety specifically? Are you a parent or grandparent? Do you need to do safety-related work in your home for a toddler or other young child visiting?

APPLYING KNOWLEDGE

1. How can you help parents deal with the fears of their toddler? Why is it important for adults to control their own fears around a toddler? If you must do an unfamiliar procedure as a student (such as giving an injection) to a toddler, how do you control your own fears?

2. How can you use assessment of expected growth and development during the toddler years or other periods of childhood to provide better care when the child is hospitalized?

3. How can parents' knowledge of a child's expected growth and development help protect the child from injury? Give examples of advice you might give to parents of an 18-month-old child, a 24-month-old child, and a 36-month-old child. If hospitalized, should you be surprised if a child's behavior becomes more like that of a younger child than the typical behavior the parent describes?

4. How does full myelination of the spinal cord relate to success of toilet training?

5. Use growth charts to determine if the physical growth of children you care for in clinical experience is normal.

6. Discuss day care with classmates who are parents. Are they satisfied with the care their children receive? What, if any, problems have they had with day care? What alternatives to day care of young children do classmates use?

The Preschool Child

chapter

18

Answer Key: A complete answer key can be found on the Student Evolve website.

LEARNING ACTIVITIES

1. Match the terms in the left column with their definitions on the right (a–e).

   _____ Animism *(421)*
   _____ Artificialism *(421)*
   _____ Centering *(421)*
   _____ Egocentrism *(421)*
   _____ Enuresis *(428)*

   a. Concentrating on a single aspect of an object
   b. Attributing lifelike qualities to inanimate objects
   c. Involuntary urination after the age at which bladder control should have been established
   d. Viewing everything in reference to oneself
   e. Belief that everything is created by people

2. State the following typical vital signs in the preschool child. *(420)*

   a. Pulse: _____ to _____ bpm

   b. Respirations: _____ breaths/minute

   c. Blood pressure: _____ systolic and _____ diastolic

3. According to Piaget, preschool-age children are in the _____ phase of cognitive development. *(421)*

4. List four characteristics of preoperational thinking. *(421)*

   a. _____

   b. _____

   c. _____

   d. _____

5. In the preschool period, the number of words in a child's sentences should equal _____
   _____. *(421)*

6. Masturbation in the preschool child is considered harmless as long as the child _____

   _____ . *(422; 424, Table 18-1)*

7. Describe the following general characteristics of the 3-year-old child. *(422-425)*

    a. Sentences are _____ than at age 2 and they can express _____ and ask _____.

    b. May have a(n) _____ attachment to the parent of the opposite sex.

8. A fear that is unique to 3-year-olds is a fear of _____ _____. *(425)*

9. Describe the following general characteristics of the 4-year-old child. *(425)*

    a. Can use _____ with success.

    b. Prefers _____ toys.

    c. Plays with friends of the _____ sex.

10. Describe the following general characteristics of the 5-year-old child. *(425-426)*

    a. At age 5, children are more _____ and have more _____.

    b. Height increases by _____ inches, and weight increases by _____ pounds.

    c. May begin losing _____ teeth.

    d. Can play games that have _____.

11. Describe three ways children benefit from having limits set on their behavior. *(426)*

    a. _____

    b. _____

    c. _____

12. Effective discipline is designed to shift responsibility for control from the _____ to the _____. *(426)*

13. Describe three discipline methods that are often effective for the preschool child. *(426-427)*

    a. _____

       _____

    b. _____

       _____

    c. _____

       _____

14. A time-out for a 3-year-old child should last _____ minutes. *(426)*

15. Thumb-sucking will not have a detrimental effect on a child's teeth if the habit is discontinued before _____. *(428)*

16. Describe the two types of enuresis. *(428)*

    a. Primary: _____

    b. Secondary: _____

17. List five possible causes of enuresis. *(428)*

    a. _____

    b. _____

    c. _____

    d. _____

    e. _____

18. The _____ age, rather than the _____ age of the intellectually disabled child should be considered when selecting toys for the child. *(431)*

19. What purpose can an imaginary friend serve for a preschool-age child? *(431)* _____

    _____

20. a. Hospitalization can be frightening to preschool children because they are _____.

    b. Their thinking is _____. *(432)*

21. Preschool children cannot fully understand cause and effect and they may perceive illness and hospitalization as _____ for past behavior. *(432)*

22. True or false?

    a. Hospitalized preschoolers may feel abandoned by their parents. *(432)* _____

    b. It would be unusual for a preschooler to have enuresis during a hospitalization. *(432)* _____

    c. Having the same nurses care for a hospitalized preschooler will lessen the stress of the experience for the child. *(432)* _____

REVIEW QUESTIONS

1. A preschool child falls off the swing and cries, "Bad swing! You made me fall!" This child's response is an example of: *(421)*
   1. egocentrism.
   2. artificialism.
   3. animism.
   4. centering.

2. Choose the best example of egocentric thinking. *(421)*
   1. "The airplane takes me to Grandma's."
   2. "Water is blue because someone colored it."
   3. "This big box is a truck."
   4. "The moon sleeps during the daytime."

3. The nurse would explain to parents that fears of preschool children are usually: *(425)*
   1. similar to those of older children.
   2. a result of the child's easy distraction.
   3. less intense than when they were younger.
   4. greater than those they had as toddlers.

4. When planning to read with a 5-year-old child, the nurse understands that favorite stories of preschool children are those that relate to their: *(425)*
   1. aggressive tendencies.
   2. self-centeredness.
   3. daily experiences.
   4. relationships with others.

5. A healthy preschool girl asks her parents if she will die. The best response is to tell her that: *(425)*
   1. people do not usually die until they are old.
   2. she does not need to worry about dying.
   3. parents usually die before their children.
   4. she will not die for a long time.

6. What is the most appropriate advice for the nurse to offer parents who are concerned about their preschooler's masturbation? *(424)*
   1. Remove the child's hands from the genitals.
   2. Try to interest the child in another activity.
   3. Tell the child not to touch himself there.
   4. Ask the child why he is rubbing that area.

7. One effective method of discipline for a preschool child is to: *(426)*
   1. reward the child for good behavior.
   2. give the child a light spanking.
   3. review the reasons for discipline.
   4. stop interacting with the child.

8. Choose the most effective way for parents to deal with a preschool child's jealousy of her new brother. *(427)*
   1. Help her choose toys to share with the new baby.
   2. Remind her of things she can do that the baby cannot.
   3. Explain that she will soon love her new brother.
   4. Ask her to share her room with the new baby at first.

9. A child who sucks his thumb is unlikely to have damage to the mouth if the thumb sucking stops before: *(428)*
   1. all deciduous teeth are erupted.
   2. speech is established.
   3. the first teeth erupt.
   4. the permanent teeth erupt.

10. Choose the most appropriate teaching for parents of a child with enuresis. *(428)*
    1. Enuresis is suggestive of emotional instability in a child.
    2. The child's fluid intake should be restricted during the day.
    3. The child should empty his bladder before going to bed.
    4. A relapse during treatment for enuresis is uncommon.

11. According to Erikson, the developmental task of the preschool period is to achieve a sense of: *(422, Table 18-1)*
    1. trust.
    2. autonomy.
    3. initiative.
    4. industry.

12. Which is the best choice for a play activity for a 4-year-old child? *(422, Table 18-1; 431)*
    1. Watch a DVD.
    2. Play a computer game.
    3. Ride a bicycle.
    4. Build with blocks.

13. Choose the approximate age when children begin playing games that have simple rules. *(422)*
    1. 3 years
    2. 4 years
    3. 5 years
    4. 6 years

14. Bedtime for the preschool child should include: *(424)*
    1. flexibility in the time the child goes to bed.
    2. a period of exercise after dinner.
    3. warm milk.
    4. a quiet activity such as a story.

15. A major cause of health problems in preschool children is: *(429)*
    1. immunization reactions.
    2. communicable diseases.
    3. environmental allergies.
    4. accidental injuries.

CASE STUDY

1. Heather is being discharged from the birth center with her second baby, a girl named Amanda. Her 3-year-old son Shawn has visited with her and Amanda for several hours since her birth. Heather expresses concern about Shawn's relationship with the new baby since he has previously been the only child in the home. What guidance should the nurse give Heather about minimizing Shawn's jealousy during the first few weeks after she and Amanda go home?

THINKING CRITICALLY

1. What are appropriate ways to encourage preschool children's desires to do things for themselves while they are hospitalized in your clinical facility?

2. How would you help parents who are concerned because their preschool child uses bad language?

APPLYING KNOWLEDGE

1. As you care for children in the clinical area, identify examples of egocentrism, animism, and artificialism in their behavior.

2. Does your clinical facility have classes for siblings when a new baby is expected? What is included in the classes?

3. What kinds of nursery schools are available in your area?
   a. Are there publicly supported nursery schools for children who are from low-income families?
   b. Is day care available onsite at the clinical facility to which you are assigned?

4. When you care for hospitalized children, are you able to use role modeling to teach parents? If you have not used role modeling, think of appropriate ways to use this parent teaching technique.

5. If your clinical facility has a play therapist, observe this staff member's work with children.

The School-Age Child

chapter
19

Answer Key: A complete answer key can be found on the Student Evolve website.

LEARNING ACTIVITIES

1. Match the terms in the left column with their definitions on the right (a–d).

   _____ Concrete operations *(434)*

   _____ Androgynous *(435)*

   _____ Latchkey child *(439, Health Promotion, Safety Alert)*

   _____ Preadolescent *(441)*

   a. Period immediately preceding adolescence

   b. Sex role concept that incorporates both masculine and feminine qualities

   c. Logical thinking and an understanding of cause and effect

   d. Unsupervised children left at home after school

2. The school-age child differs from the preschool child in that he or she is more interested in _____ than in fantasy. *(434)*

3. According to Erikson, the school-age period is referred to as the stage of _____. *(435, Box 19-1)*

4. Concrete operations involve _____ thinking and an understanding of _____ and _____. *(434)*

5. School-age children prefer friends of the _____ sex. *(435, Box 19-1)*

6. Give approximate growth and vital sign ranges for the school-age child. *(435; 444, Table 19-3)*

   a. Average weight gain: _____ kg/year; _____ pounds/year

   b. Average increase in height: _____cm/year; _____ inches/year

   c. Pulse: _____ to _____ bpm

   d. Respiratory rate: _____ to _____ breaths/minute

   e. Systolic blood pressure: _____ to _____ mm Hg

   f. Diastolic blood pressure: _____ to _____ mm Hg

7. How would the nurse advise parents to answer the school-age child's questions about sex? *(436)*

   _____

   _____

8. Describe information school-age children need in preparation for puberty. *(436)*

    a. Boys: _____

    _____

    b. Girls: _____

    _____

9. True or false?

    a. Belonging to a group is important to school-age children. *(437, Table 19-2)* _____

    b. Latchkey children are at higher risk for accidents. *(439; Health Promotion, Safety Alert)* _____

10. Describe the following typical characteristics of a 6-year-old child. *(439-440)*

    a. The attention span is _____.

    b. Loss of _____ teeth occurs, along with eruption of

    _____.

    c. Greater exposure to _____ occurs with entry into school.

    d. Needs _____ hours of sleep per night.

11. The 7-year-old child prefers toys that are _____

    _____. *(440)*

12. Describe the following typical characteristics of an 8-year-old child. *(440)*

    a. Prefers friends of the _____ sex.

    b. What type of sports does this child enjoy? _____ How does the 8-year-old take loss of a game? _____

    c. Secret clubs have strict _____.

13. Describe the following typical characteristics of a 9-year-old child. *(440-441, Fig. 19-6)*

    a. Common behaviors of the 9-year-old that may indicate tension include _____ and

    _____.

    b. What type of sports and other recreational activities are popular for 9-year-olds? _____

    _____

    _____

    c. Needs _____ hours of sleep per night.

14. Describe the following typical characteristics of a 10-year-old preadolescent. *(441-442)*

    a. Strives for _____, but will take suggestions.

    b. Ideas of the _____ are more important than those of the individual.

    c. Takes greater interest in his or her _____.

15. Describe the behavior changes of 11- and 12-year-old preadolescents. *(442)*

    a. This period is one of complete _____.

    b. Less ability to _____ can cause school grades to decline.

    c. The child has _____ permanent teeth.

16. What type of atmosphere should the parents of a school-age child create for doing homework? *(443)*

    _____

    _____

17. True or false? *(443, 447)*

    a. Children with an allergy to animal dander should not have a pet. _____

    b. Children older than 7 years can be responsible for caring for a pet. _____

    c. Having a pet can foster a sense of responsibility and encourage socialization for a shy child. _____

REVIEW QUESTIONS

1. The school-age child who has few experiences of success is likely to develop a sense of: *(434)*
   1. dependence.
   2. inferiority.
   3. trust.
   4. industry.

2. Which best describes physical growth of the school-age child? *(434)*
   1. Rapid growth occurs from 6–9 years of age and then slows.
   2. Slow growth continues until just before puberty.
   3. Height increases faster than weight.
   4. Height and weight remain stable until the onset of puberty.

3. Choose the normal characteristics of vital signs that the nurse should expect when assessing a 9-year-old girl. *(435)*
   1. Blood pressure and pulse are higher than those of boys the same age.
   2. Blood pressure, pulse, and respirations are close to adult levels.
   3. Blood pressure is higher, but pulse and respirations are lower than the adult.
   4. Blood pressure, pulse, and respirations are higher than those of a 6-year-old girl.

4. How would the nurse advise parents regarding a school-age child's questions about sex? *(436)*
   1. Initiate discussions before the child asks any questions.
   2. Answer questions at the child's level of understanding.
   3. Assure parents the topic will be part of the school curriculum.
   4. Select terms that are used by school-age children.

5. The most significant physical development at age 6 years is: *(439-440)*
   1. loss of the primary teeth.
   2. round, moon-shaped face.
   3. better infection resistance.
   4. rapid growth in height.

6. Worries and minor compulsions are more common at the age of: *(441)*
   1. 6 years.
   2. 7 years.
   3. 9 years.
   4. 11 years.

7. A preadolescent is more likely to accept her parents' decision if: *(442)*
   1. she understands why her parents made the decision.
   2. the parents do not change decisions once they are made.
   3. the parents carefully control the child's friends.
   4. her friends have values similar to her own family's.

8. Which statement made by a 10-year-old child indicates the need for teaching about living a healthy life-style? *(444-445; Table 19-3)*
   1. "I go to the dentist twice a year."
   2. "I wear a helmet when I ride my bike."
   3. "I watch 4 hours of television after school."
   4. "I go to bed at 9:00 PM and get up at 7:00 AM."

9. The preadolescent girl should have supplies for menstruation: *(436; 446, Table 19-3)*
   1. before her first menstrual period.
   2. as soon as she knows how heavy her flow is.
   3. when her friends are prepared for theirs.
   4. about 6 months after breast development begins.

10. A group of 8- and 9-year-old boys has formed a "club." The boys have a secret password and handshake before they meet. Parents should interpret this behavior as: *(438; 445, Table 19-3)*
    1. typical for children in this age group.
    2. a way to avoid being around adults.
    3. preceding criminal-type gang membership.
    4. rebellion against bossy older children.

11. A father is concerned because his 9-year-old son has developed the habit of wrinkling his nose uncon-sciously. The nurse should tell the father that his son: *(441)*
    1. may have a nerve problem and should be seen by a physician.
    2. cannot get adequate adult attention without taking this action.
    3. is probably doing this because of unresolved tension.
    4. should be corrected any time he is caught doing this action.

12. A school-age child has an adult "hero" of the same sex. What is the most appropriate interpretation of this behavior? *(434, 440)*
    1. The child feels insecure and inadequate around other children.
    2. Identifying with adults of the same sex is common at this time.
    3. Molestation or sexual abuse by the adult should be considered.
    4. The child is exploring various career and lifestyle options.

13. Which statement characterizes the 8-year-old child? *(440)*
    1. Eight-year-olds are totally disorganized.
    2. They are beginning to take an increased interest in their appearance.
    3. At this age, children are quieter and more modest than the year before.
    4. They like competitive sports, but are poor losers.

CASE STUDIES

1. Becca, 6 years old, is receiving her booster immunizations before starting school. Her mother tells you that she is concerned about how Becca will adjust to school because it is the first time she will be away from home for a significant part of the day. How can you help her mother prepare Becca for school?

2. Logan, 10 years old, is hospitalized in skeletal traction with a badly fractured wrist and humerus that he suffered when playing street hockey with his friends. Logan says he is really unhappy about being away from his friends during summer vacation. The boys spend most of the warm hours of the day at the public pool and either skate or ride their bikes until dark. What safety teaching does Logan need? How can you use knowledge of preadolescent growth and development to teach Logan and his family about safety? What can you do to meet his needs for companionship with his friends?

THINKING CRITICALLY

1. For each category listed below, describe one or two ways the nurse can incorporate the needs of the school-age child into care during hospitalization.
   a. Encouraging decision-making
   b. Need for inclusion in a group

APPLYING KNOWLEDGE

1. Observe how nurses experienced in pediatrics prepare children of different ages for medical procedures. Identify ways they use knowledge of growth and development when caring for children of different ages, but with similar medical conditions.

2. Watch popular television programs and evaluate them critically for positive and potentially harmful influences on children. Consider the following factors:
   a. Stimulating the child's imagination
   b. Materialistic focus
   c. Stereotypes (gender, age, race, and family structure)
   d. Violent content

3. Check at your clinical facility for availability of pet therapy. If this therapy is available, how is it used to achieve the therapeutic goal?

The Adolescent

Answer Key: A complete answer key can be found on the Student Evolve website.

LEARNING ACTIVITIES

1. Match the terms in the left column with their definitions on the right (a–g).

   _____ Adolescence *(450)*

   _____ Androgens *(451)*

   _____ Estrogens *(451)*

   _____ Menarche *(453)*

   _____ Puberty *(451)*

   _____ Growth spurt *(451)*

   _____ Self-concept *(453, Table 20-1; 456, Box 20-1)*

   a. One's view of oneself
   b. Rapid period of growth in which the body reaches adult height and weight
   c. First menstrual period
   d. Period during which reproductive organs become functional
   e. Female sex hormones
   f. Male sex hormones
   g. Period beginning with appearance of secondary sex characteristics and ending with physical and emotional maturity

2. List the four major tasks of adolescence. *(450)*

   a. _____

   b. _____

   c. _____

   d. _____

3. In the formal operations stage of cognitive development, late adolescents are capable of _____ reasoning. *(451)*

4. One of the strongest needs of adolescents is _____. *(451)*

5. Define *preadolescence*. *(451)*_____

   _____

6. Puberty occurs earlier in which gender? _____ *(451)*

7. The first change of puberty in a boy is _____ _____. *(451)*

8. Boys begin sperm production at about _____ years of age. *(453)*

9. Two important cancer detection tests that are appropriately taught during adolescence are the monthly _____ and _____ self-examinations. *(456, Nursing Tip)*

10. Erikson identifies the major task of adolescence as _____. *(456, Nursing Tip)*

11. Describe several possible adult outcomes if the adolescent does not achieve his or her own identity. *(456)*

   _____

   _____

   _____

   _____

12. True or false? *(457)*

   a. Adolescents think everyone is looking at them. _____

   b. An adolescent's preoccupation with his or her appearance is a normal behavior. _____

13. How can cliques facilitate adolescent peer relationships? *(457)* _____

   _____

14. State ways parents can help their teenager develop increased responsibility in each of the following areas. *(456)*

   a. Routine tasks: _____

   _____

   _____

   b. Managing money: _____

   _____

   _____

15. True or false?

   a. Daydreaming is a warning sign of a mental health problem. *(459)* _____

   b. An adolescent's cultural background can influence dating behavior. *(459)* _____

   c. Sexual curiosity and masturbation are common among adolescents. *(459)* _____

   d. Parents should answer an adolescent's questions about sex truthfully. *(460)* _____

   e. Sexual experimentation with same-sex partners during adolescence is a predictor of homosexuality. *(460)* _____

16. List two factors that increase the risk for nutritional deficiencies during adolescence. *(462)*

   a. _____

   _____

   b. _____

   _____

17. An adolescent's diet is most likely to be deficient in which three nutrients? *(462)*

    a. _____

    b. _____

    c. _____

18. An adolescent who follows a vegan diet should be advised to include foods that provide sufficient quantities of which nutrients? *(463)*

    a. _____

    b. _____

    c. _____

    d. _____

    e. _____

    f. _____

19. Use of a(n) _____ is the primary safety risk for an adolescent. *(464)*

20. High school students who participate in competitive sports should have a comprehensive _____ screening. *(464)*

21. A change in school performance, appearance, and behavior can be a warning sign of _____. *(465)*

REVIEW QUESTIONS

1. Younger adolescents often have an awkward appearance because: *(451)*
   1. maturation occurs earlier than in previous generations.
   2. body parts grow and mature at different rates.
   3. growth and development slows during adolescence.
   4. self-consciousness causes the adolescent to slump.

2. A person who does not establish an identity during adolescence is more likely to: *(456)*
   1. become a little too flexible in establishing rules or boundaries.
   2. conform to a peer group for a prolonged time.
   3. have an overly superior self-image.
   4. become fearful of changes.

3. A parent can best help an adolescent make a wise decision by: *(456, Nursing Tip)*
   1. explaining what he or she would have done when he or she was a teenager.
   2. reviewing problems with the decision after the teenager makes it.
   3. serving as a role model by making the decision for the teenager.
   4. respecting the teenager's decision, even if he or she makes a mistake.

4. Younger adolescents tend to be egocentric because they are: *(457)*
   1. certain that their parents are ignorant.
   2. believe no-one is paying attention to them.
   3. preoccupied with their physical development.
   4. proud of their greater responsibilities.

5. The adolescent's peer group helps him or her move away from: *(457, Fig. 20-8)*
   1. same-sex friendships.
   2. values of his or her family.
   3. individual responsibility.
   4. dependence on his or her family.

6. What is the best nursing response to a parent who is concerned about her 15-year-old's frequent day-dreaming? *(459)*
   1. "Daydreaming is a normal adolescent occurrence."
   2. "This behavior is an indicator of adolescent insecurity."
   3. "Your concern is valid because this is a sign of depression."
   4. "It is a way for teenagers to ignore their parents."

7. An adolescent who adopts a strict vegetarian diet is at risk for a deficiency of which nutrient? *(463)*
   1. Carbohydrates
   2. Vitamin C
   3. Protein
   4. Fiber

8. Most accidents involving adolescents occur when they: *(464)*
   1. participate in contact sports.
   2. handle guns or knives.
   3. drive a car or other vehicle.
   4. work at part-time jobs.

9. The nurse assessing an adolescent's physical development knows that the Tanner stages describe the: *(454, Box 20-2)*
   1. sequence of physical maturation in the adolescent.
   2. change from concrete thinking to abstract thinking.
   3. hormonal changes that cause ovulation and menstruation.
   4. development of a mature gender identity.

10. The major psychosocial task of adolescence is to develop a sense of: *(450)*
    1. sexual orientation.
    2. concern for other people.
    3. family unity.
    4. identity as an individual.

11. A parent is worried because her 14-year-old son seems to be constantly in the bathroom, shampooing and styling his hair. She worries that her son may be homosexual because he is so concerned about his appearance. What is the most appropriate nursing response to the mother's concern? *(457)*
    1. "Homosexual thoughts and experimentation are normal during the early teens."
    2. "Boys are usually more concerned about their athletic abilities than their appearance."
    3. "You should be more concerned about why he does not want to be with his friends."
    4. "Teens are preoccupied with their appearance because of dramatic body changes."

12. What is the best information for the nurse to include in a class for adolescents about healthy eating habits? *(462)*
    1. How to choose foods from MyPlate, provided by the FDA.
    2. The need to eat three balanced meals per day.
    3. The importance of an adequate diet to better health during adulthood.
    4. Nutrients that are often lacking in an adolescent's diet.

13. What is the best food choice for an adolescent who just finished playing a game of field hockey? *(463)*
    1. Cheese slice
    2. Chocolate bar
    3. Garden salad
    4. Toasted bagel

CASE STUDIES

1. Austin's mother is worried about the change for the worse in the behavior of her only child who is 14 years old. "Our family has always enjoyed many activities together, but now Austin only wants to be with his friends. He doesn't seem to care that his clothes look bizarre, and yet he's constantly fussing with his hair. He never seems to pay attention. I'm afraid his grades will fall and he won't get into a good college." What advice can you offer Austin's mother to help her understand her son's behavior?

2. Megan, 15 years old, confides to you that she and her boyfriend have had sex a few times. Megan is concerned about getting pregnant, but does not know much about contraception. She says that talking to her parents about sex and contraception is out of the question.
    a. How can you help Megan make responsible decisions concerning her sexuality?
    b. What problems have you seen in adolescents who become parents?

THINKING CRITICALLY

1. A 15-year-old girl is at the pediatrician's office for a well-child examination. After you measure her weight, she tells you she is worried about being fat. Her weight is at the 75th percentile for her age. How would you respond to the girl's comment?

2. You are assigned to care for a 14-year-old boy. He responds to your questions with one-word answers. What strategies would you use to establish a rapport with this adolescent?

APPLYING KNOWLEDGE

1. Observe a group of young adolescents. Identify behaviors in the group that demonstrate the following:
    a. Efforts to develop an identity
    b. Preoccupation with self
    c. Cultural variations

2. Obtain the most recent national statistics for motor vehicle accidents (MVA) involving teenagers. See http://www.cdc.gov/Motorvehiclesafety/ and local or state statistical websites.
    a. How long have most teens who have MVAs been licensed?
    b. What is the incidence of alcohol abuse in teens and how does this compare to adults cited for driving under the influence?
    c. Were cell phones or texting involved?
    d. What is the fatality rate for MVAs involving teens?

3. Visit community groups that focus on reducing gang violence among teenagers. Determine the approximate ages of gang members and how they identify themselves to one another and to rival gangs.

4. Obtain local statistics for violent deaths among teenagers. How many of these are thought to be related to gangs?

The Child's Experience of Hospitalization

chapter

21

Answer Key: A complete answer key can be found on the Student Evolve website.

LEARNING ACTIVITIES

1. Match the terms in the left column with their definitions on the right (a–d).

   _____ Clinical pathway *(478)*

   _____ Emancipated minor *(483)*

   _____ Regression *(474)*

   _____ Respite care *(484)*

   a. Trained workers come to the home to relieve parents
   b. Loss of an achieved level of functioning to a past level of behavior
   c. Interdisciplinary plan of care that displays progress of the treatment plan for a patient
   d. Adolescent younger than 18 years of age who is no longer under the parents' authority

2. List three or more advantages of outpatient surgery for the child. *(469)*

   a. _____

   b. _____

   c. _____

3. What age-appropriate nursing strategies are useful to prepare a 3-year-old for a procedure? Include average attention span for 3-year-olds. *(Box 21-1, 470, Table 18-1)*

   _____

   _____

   _____

4. A child's reaction to hospitalization depends on which factors? *(470)*

   a. _____

   b. _____

   c. _____

   d. _____

   e. _____

   f. _____

5. True or false?

   a. Every child reacts differently to the hospital experience. *(470)* _____

   b. During hospitalization, a caring and compassionate nurse can take the place of a child's primary caregivers. *(470-471)* _____

   c. Hospitalization can be a positive experience for children. *(471)* _____

6. What are the three major stressors for children of all ages during hospitalization? *(471)*

   a. _____

   b. _____

   c. _____

7. Separation anxiety is most pronounced in the _____ age group. *(471)*

8. Match the stage of separation anxiety with the behavior that corresponds with the stage (a–c). *(471-472, Nursing Tip)*

   _____ Protest   a. Child is sad and depressed.
   _____ Despair   b. Child becomes interested in his or her surroundings.
   _____ Denial   c. Child cries continuously for "mommy."

9. Assessment of pain is recorded when _____. *(472)*

10. Describe three or more nonpharmacologic methods of pain reduction. Have you used any of these methods for yourself or your child? Did the method or methods have the desired effect? *(472)*

    a. _____

    b. _____

    c. _____

11. Administration of acetaminophen in quantities exceeding the recommended maximum daily dose can cause damage to the _____. *(474)*

12. True or false? *(474)*

    a. Infants and children respond to drugs differently than adults. _____

    b. Addiction occurs quickly in children receiving opioids for severe pain. _____

    c. Children 7 years of age and older can be taught to use patient-controlled analgesia. _____

    d. Administering analgesics on an as-needed schedule is the most effective way to relieve a child's pain. _____

    e. The nurse must calculate all medication dosages to determine if they are safe to administer to the child. _____

13. Define *conscious sedation*. *(474)* _____

14. What advice would the nurse give to a parent who is concerned that her hospitalized toddler was drinking from a cup and now only wants his bottle? *(474-475)*

_____

_____

15. Describe three or more things the nurse can do to lessen anxiety for the parents of a hospitalized child. *(475, Nursing Care Plan 21-1; 476; 477, Nursing Tip)*

a. _____

_____

b. _____

_____

c. _____

_____

16. Describe two ways the nurse can decrease siblings' anxiety when a brother or sister is hospitalized. *(477)*

a. _____

_____

b. _____

_____

17. List five or more topics that are included in a developmental history. Describe how you would assess and/or describe each of the five. *(478)*

a. _____

b. _____

c. _____

d. _____

e. _____

18. List two methods of decreasing the stress of hospitalization for an infant. *(479-480)*

a. _____

b. _____

19. List three examples of transitional objects that can be brought to the hospital for a 15-month-old child. *(480, Box 21-2)*

a. _____

b. _____

c. _____

20. What guidelines should the nurse follow for providing explanations about hospital experiences to young children? *(479-480; Box 21-2)*

    a. _____

    b. _____

    c. _____

21. Preschoolers are particularly fearful of _____. *(481)*

22. Explain how the nurse would prepare a preschool child for abdominal surgery. *(481)* _____

    _____

23. Describe two or more ways the nurse can foster a sense of independence for the hospitalized school-age child. *(482)*

    a. _____

    b. _____

24. Following treatments, what should the nurse encourage the school-age child to do? *(482, Safety Alert)*

    _____

25. Illness in the young adolescent is perceived mainly as a threat to _____ _____. *(482)*

26. What factors should the nurse take into consideration when assigning rooms or roommates for a hospitalized adolescent? *(483)*

    _____

    _____

27. a. Preparation for discharge begins _____. *(483)*

    b. How does pediatric discharge preparation compare to discharge for adults that you may have done?

       _____

       _____

       _____

28. What should be included in the documentation when a child is discharged from the hospital? How does this compare to the documentation you have done for an adult or a mother and her newborn? *(483-484)*

    a. _____

    b. _____

    c. _____

    d. _____

    e. _____

29. List four suggestions the nurse can give parents who are concerned about behavioral problems arising with their children after hospitalization. *(483)*

    a. _____

    b. _____

    c. _____

    d. _____

REVIEW QUESTIONS

1. Separation anxiety is most pronounced in which age group? *(471)*
   1. Infants
   2. Toddlers
   3. Preschool children
   4. Adolescents

2. The mother of a hospitalized toddler could best explain when she will return by saying, "I will be back: *(480)*
   1. in 3 hours."
   2. after your nap."
   3. before six o'clock."
   4. before you know it."

3. In most instances, unpleasant treatments on children should take place in the: *(471)*
   1. playroom.
   2. emergency department.
   3. child's room.
   4. treatment room.

4. Which child is most likely to feel his or her illness is punishment for something he or she has done wrong? *(481)*
   1. Toddler
   2. Preschool
   3. School-age
   4. Adolescent

5. Which intervention is most appropriate to reduce a 5-year-old's anxiety related to upcoming surgery? *(470)*
   1. Do not tell the child that he or she is having surgery.
   2. Arrange for the child to meet the surgeon.
   3. Schedule a visit to the surgical area preoperatively.
   4. Give the child a ride on the stretcher before surgery.

6. Parental consent for minors is not always necessary for treatment in which situation? *(483)*
   1. Minor cuts and abrasions
   2. Psychologic disorders
   3. Communicable diseases
   4. Sexually transmitted infections

7. The mother of a 3-year-old child is concerned because he has returned to diapers since he has been hospitalized although he had been potty trained. What is the best nursing response to the mother? *(474-475)*
    1. "This is unusual and probably temporary."
    2. "Keep him in his training pants and don't give in to him."
    3. "Regression is normal in a sick child."
    4. "Perhaps he has some type of urinary infection."

8. The nurse's best approach to prepare a toddler for a painful procedure is to: *(480)*
    1. be truthful if it will be painful.
    2. avoid telling him it might hurt.
    3. prepare early so he can ask questions.
    4. have his mother explain what will happen.

9. What action would the nurse take when a hospitalized school-age child begins to act out? *(482)*
    1. Place the child in a private room.
    2. Discipline the child by having restrictions put in place.
    3. Provide positive direction and consistency.
    4. Ignore the behavior because this is an expected reaction.

10. After performing a painful procedure on an infant, the nurse should: *(479)*
    1. swaddle the infant.
    2. feed the infant.
    3. return the infant to the parent.
    4. change the infant's diaper.

11. The nurse would expect a common reaction to hospitalization for a 4-year-old child to be: *(481)*
    1. anger.
    2. depression.
    3. guilt.
    4. fear.

12. The nurse understands that a hospitalized school-age child should be allowed to participate in his or her own care in order to: *(482)*
    1. decrease fear of bodily injury.
    2. increase self-esteem.
    3. allow some control.
    4. reduce responsibility.

13. What is the best nursing approach to decrease a preschooler's anxiety about having his blood pressure measured? *(480)*
    1. Take the blood pressure while the child is sleeping.
    2. Ask the child's mother to take the blood pressure.
    3. Demonstrate the procedure on a doll prior to performing it on the child.
    4. Tell the child that big boys and girls do not cry when they have their blood pressure taken.

14. A child is receiving morphine sulfate for pain management after an inguinal hernia repair. What is the most appropriate response to parents who are concerned their child will become addicted to the medication? *(474)*
    1. "Addiction to narcotics is rare in children."
    2. "Is there a family history of drug addiction?"
    3. "The dosage is insufficient to produce addiction."
    4. "This is the best medication to control your child's pain."

15. An 18-month-old child has been crying for "mommy" since the parent left several hours ago. How would the nurse interpret the toddler's behavior? *(471-472, Nursing Care Plan 21-1; 475)*
    1. This is the child's first separation from his mother.
    2. The child is experiencing separation anxiety.
    3. The illness is causing the child to have severe pain.
    4. The child is detached from his father.

CASE STUDY

1. Connor, 15 months old, is admitted to the hospital with a diagnosis of croup. Both of his parents work and care for two older siblings. (See also Chapter 25 for information about croup.)
   a. What factors will affect Connor's reaction to hospitalization?
   b. What information will you collect in a developmental history?
   c. How will you use this information to provide nursing care to this toddler?
   d. Connor's mother confides to the nurse that she feels that this hospitalization could have been avoided if she would have taken Connor to the doctor sooner. How can you best answer the mother?
   e. Following admission to the pediatric unit, Connor's parents leave to make arrangements for their other children. Connor cries continuously for his mother. What is your interpretation of this behavior?
   f. Connor's 5-year-old sister asks you if her little brother is going to die like when her grandfather was in the hospital. How should you respond to this question?

THINKING CRITICALLY

1. Prepare a care plan for a hospitalized toddler. Address the psychosocial needs of the child and parents. Include nursing diagnoses, goals, and interventions.

2. Do you think parents have the right to know if their children are being treated for a sexually transmitted infection? How does your position on parental knowledge compare with current recommendations to start human papillomavirus (HPV) vaccinations? Discuss these issues with your classmates.

APPLYING KNOWLEDGE

1. Involve a school-age child in a board game. How effective was this strategy with establishing rapport and communication with the child?

2. While you are in the clinical area, assess a toddler who is alone for signs of separation anxiety. What stage of separation anxiety corresponds to the child's behaviors?

3. Take a hospitalized child to the playroom. Compare the child's behavior while in the playroom to behavior in the hospital room.

4. Discuss with your peers how you feel when parents do not come to visit their hospitalized child. What could be some reasons for their not visiting?

5. Determine the laws in your state governing the treatment of minors.

Health Care Adaptations for the Child and Family

Answer Key: A complete answer key can be found on the Student Evolve website.

LEARNING ACTIVITIES

1. Match the terms in the left column with their definitions on the right (a–d).

   _____ Auscultation *(491)*
   _____ Parenteral fluids *(506)*
   _____ Saline lock *(506)*
   _____ TPN *(506)*

   a. A device to keep a vein open for intermittent medication administration
   b. Given by a route other than the digestive tract
   c. Hyperalimentation
   d. Blood pressure assessment with stethoscope and blood pressure cuff

2. What is implied when a parent or guardian gives his or her written informed consent for a child to receive medical treatment? *(486)*

   _____

   _____

3. A consent form must be signed by the _____, the _____, and a(n) _____. *(486)*

4. The nurse acts as a(n) _____ _____ in ensuring proper consent has been signed _____ a procedure and that the child is given an age-appropriate explanation of the procedure. *(486)*

5. List at least six safety measures applicable to the hospitalized child. Place a star beside any safety measure that would apply equally to a child and older teen or adult. *(487; Safety Alert)*

   a. _____

   _____

   b. _____

   _____

   c. _____

   _____

   d. _____

   _____

   e. _____

   _____

   f. _____

   _____

6. Describe four or more safety hazards to avoid when caring for a hospitalized child. *(487)*

   a. _____

   _____

   b. _____

   _____

   c. _____

   _____

   d. _____

   _____

7. Identify three factors the nurse must consider when selecting the method for transporting a child from the pediatric unit to the radiology department. *(488)*

   a. _____

   b. _____

   c. _____

8. Name two procedures for which the nurse might use a mummy restraint for an infant. *(488; 489, Skill 22-1)*

   a. _____

   b. _____

9. What is the purpose of the personal history survey? *(490)* _____

   _____

   _____

10. True or false?

    a. Bradycardia is often the first sign of shock in infants and children. *(491)* _____

    b. Hypotension is an early sign of shock in children. *(490)* _____

    c. Bradycardia is considered a medical emergency in infants and young children. *(491)* _____

    d. Medication dosages in children are determined by the child's weight. *(491)* _____

11. A(n) _____ fontanelle may indicate dehydration and a(n) _____ fontanelle may indicate increased intracranial pressure. *(491)*

12. Apical pulses are advised for children under age _____ years and should be counted for _____ seconds. *(491)*

13. The width of the blood pressure cuff should cover _____ of the upper arm. *(492)*

14. *Fever* is defined as a temperature (a) over _____°C/_____°F for rectal or tympanic or (b) over _____°C/_____°F for axillary. *(494; 496, Nursing Care Plan 22-1)*

15. Why is it important to obtain an accurate weight measurement for infants and young children? *(491)*

_____

_____

16. To accurately measure the temperature of a 4-year-old child using a tympanic thermometer, the nurse would gently pull the pinna (earlobe) _____ and _____. *(495, Skill 22-4)*

17. Describe the procedure for weighing an infant. *(495)* _____

_____

_____

_____

_____

18. Describe the procedure for collecting a urine specimen from an infant. *(498, Skill 22-5)* _____

_____

_____

_____

_____

19. What is the purpose of a lumbar puncture? *(498)* _____

_____

_____

20. a.   Explain how a nurse should position a 10-year-old child for a lumbar puncture. *(499; Fig. 22-7A)*

_____

_____

_____

   b.   Describe the correct position to use for a 12-month-old infant having a lumbar puncture. *(499; Fig. 22-7B)* _____

_____

_____

21. What information should be recorded after a lumbar puncture? *(499)* _____

_____

_____

_____

22. _____ is the most important variable in predicting response to any drug therapy. *(500)*

23. Why are drugs metabolized more slowly by infants and young children? *(500)* _____

_____

24. Describe the procedure for administering medication to an infant with an oral syringe. *(508, Box 22-1; 501, Skill 22-6)*

_____

_____

_____

25. Compare the procedure for administering ear drops to children younger than 3 years of age and children 3 years of age and older. *(502; 503, Skill 22-8)*

_____

_____

_____

_____

_____

26. a.   Which site would the nurse use to administer an intramuscular injection to a 6-month-old infant? *(503, Medication Safety Alert)*

_____

   b.   Why is this the preferred site? _____

_____

27. The maximum volume that can be injected in one site for infants is _____. *(503, Medication Safety Alert)*

28. IV medications can cause _____, and the nurse must observe the child's IV site every _____ for signs of _____. *(505)*

29. How frequently does the nurse assess a child's intravenous infusion? *(505)* _____

30. Total parenteral nutrition is given to children who _____
_____. *(506)*

31. What is the appropriate nursing action when the nurse observes brown fluid draining from an infant's gastrostomy tube? *(513; Skill 22-10)*

_____

_____

_____

32. Describe the procedure for suctioning a child with a tracheostomy. *(516)* _____

_____

_____

_____

_____

_____

_____

_____

33. List five signs that might indicate a problem in a tracheostomy patient. *(517)*

a. _____

b. _____

c. _____

d. _____

e. _____

34. What emergency equipment should be kept at the bedside of a tracheostomy patient? *(517)*

_____

_____

35. What information should be included in the documentation when assessing a child with a tracheostomy? *(517)*

a. _____

b. _____

c. _____

d. _____

e. _____

36. Prior to surgery, infants should not be maintained on NPO status longer than _____ to _____ hours because of the risk of _____. *(520; Tables 22-9 and 22-10)*

REVIEW QUESTIONS

1. The nurse is aware of which variation in pulse and respiration rates of children as compared to adults? *(491)*
   1. Lower than adults
   2. Same rates as adults
   3. Higher than adults
   4. Lower at birth, but higher by age 3 years

2.   Which is the preferred way to counteract the effects of an unpleasant-tasting medication? *(501, Skill 22-6)*
     1.   Let the child choose whether to mix it with a food or not.
     2.   Mix the medication with formula or milk only so that it isn't skipped.
     3.   Follow with an "ice pop" chaser.
     4.   Mix with something thick like applesauce.

3.   An infant's diaper weighs 30 g. How many milliliters would the nurse record on the intake and output sheet? *(513, Skill 22-5; 513, Nursing Tip on diaper weight)*
     1.   15
     2.   30
     3.   45
     4.   60

4.   When caring for a tracheostomy patient, the nurse would: *(516)*
     1.   limit suctioning to no more than 15 seconds.
     2.   apply suction as the catheter is being inserted.
     3.   use a suction catheter that is approximately the same diameter as the tracheotomy tube.
     4.   replace the suction catheter and water used to clear the catheter at the end of the shift.

5.   A child weighing 35.5 pounds has an oral medication ordered at 8:00 AM. The recommended pediatric dosage is 3–5 mg/kg for the ordered drug. A safe dosage for this child would be: *(509)*
     1.   75 mg.
     2.   105 mg.
     3.   150 mg.
     4.   200 mg.

6.   What is the best way for the nurse to weigh an infant? *(495)*
     1.   Completely naked
     2.   Wearing a dry diaper
     3.   Wrapped in a receiving blanket
     4.   Lightly dressed

7.   The neonate exposed to prolonged high oxygen concentrations is at risk for damage to which part of the body? *(517)*
     1.   Heart
     2.   Eyes
     3.   Brain
     4.   Kidneys

8.   The nurse assessing a child's vital signs would count both the pulse and respirations for _____ seconds. *(491)*
     1.   15
     2.   30
     3.   45
     4.   60

9.   The nurse planning to measure a child's blood pressure would choose a cuff that covers: *(492)*
     1.   one-half of the upper arm.
     2.   one-third of the upper arm.
     3.   two-thirds of the upper arm.
     4.   the entire upper arm.

10. A 4-month-old infant's pulse rate is 140 beats per minute. How would the nurse interpret this assessment finding? *(491, Table 22-1)*
    1. Within normal limits
    2. Tachycardia
    3. Bradycardia
    4. Life-threatening situation

11. The preferred intramuscular injection site for infants is the: *(503, Fig 22-9)*
    1. deltoid.
    2. ventrogluteal.
    3. vastus lateralis.
    4. dorsogluteal.

12. The maximum volume that can be given by intramuscular injection at one site to a 3-week-old infant is: *(503, Medication Safety Alert)*
    1. 0.1 mL.
    2. 0.5 mL.
    3. 1.0 mL.
    4. 1.5 mL.

13. An expectant parent tells the nurse, "I am planning to put the baby in an antique crib." What advice on crib safety would the nurse offer to this parent? *(488, Safety Alert)*
    1. The crib slats should be no more than 2⅜ inches apart.
    2. Measure the crib slats to be sure they are at least 2⅜ inches wide.
    3. There should be 2⅜ inches between the mattress and the side rail.
    4. Keep the side rails 2⅜ inches higher than the baby's length.

14. After administering a gastrostomy tube feeding, how would the nurse position an infant? *(515, Skill 22-10)*
    1. Left side
    2. Supine
    3. Right side
    4. Prone

15. The nurse appropriately positions a 7-year-old child for a lumbar puncture: *(499, Fig 22-7A)*
    1. prone with knees flexed to the chest.
    2. lying on the side in a fetal position.
    3. sitting up and hugging the nurse.
    4. supine with the head flexed to the chest.

16. The nurse explained to a parent the procedure for administering an oral antibiotic to an infant. Which statement made by the parent indicates a correct understanding of the information? *(502)*
    1. "I should use a syringe with a short, thin needle."
    2. "Put the medicine in a bottle with a small amount of water."
    3. "Use an oral syringe to place the medicine in the side of the mouth."
    4. "Bring the medicine cup to the baby's lips to drink slowly."

17. What is the most appropriate nursing intervention to prepare a 4-year-old child for placement of an intravenous line? *(511, Table 22-5)*
    1. Tell the child that he needs the IV a few hours before the procedure.
    2. Provide an explanation for why he needs to have an IV.
    3. Let the child know that crying is okay when something hurts.
    4. Show the child the mummy restraint that will be used.

THINKING CRITICALLY

1. You are assisting a registered nurse who is going to start intravenous fluids on a 3-month-old infant. The mother is crying and is not sure if she wants to be with the infant or to remain outside the room during the procedure. How could you support this mother?

2. A physician ordered oral amoxicillin 0.25 grams every 12 hours. The pharmacy provides a bottle labeled amoxicillin 500 mg per 5 mL. Use the dimensional analysis formula to calculate and state the volume of medication the nurse should give.

3. A physician orders 500 mg oral amoxicillin solution every 12 hours for a 3-year-old girl's otitis media (ear infection). She weighed 33 pounds when she arrived at the clinic. The daily recommended dose for amoxicillin by Centers for Disease Control and Prevention (CDC) and American Academy of Pediatrics (AAP) is 80–90 mg/kg/day given in 2–3 divided doses. Make these calculations:
    a. Calculate the child's weight in kilograms.
    b. Calculate the recommended milligrams of amoxicillin for each dose.
    c. Does the ordered dose of 500 mg every 12 hours meet the recommendation?
    d. Is this ordered dose safe to give the child?
    e. Does the dose ordered in question 2 meet the current recommended dose for a 3-year-old?

APPLYING KNOWLEDGE

1. Where would the following items and areas be found in the clinical setting?
    a. Blood pressure machine
    b. Diapers
    c. Emergency cart
    d. Intake and output sheet
    e. IV set
    f. Oral medication syringe
    g. Playroom
    h. Procedure manual
    i. Scales
    j. Thermometer
    k. Treatment room
    l. Urine collection bag

2. Assist a registered nurse when she starts an IV on a child.

3. Care for a child with a tracheotomy.

4. Care for a child receiving gastrostomy tube feedings.

5. Care for a child with an IV infusing.

The Child with a Sensory or Neurological Condition

Answer Key: A complete answer key can be found on the Student Evolve website.

LEARNING ACTIVITIES

1. Match the terms in the left column with their definitions on the right (a–j).

   _____ Enucleation *(533)*
   _____ Hyperopia *(530)*
   _____ Myringotomy *(527)*
   _____ Nystagmus *(538)*
   _____ Papilledema *(538)*
   _____ Postictal lethargy *(541)*
   _____ Strabismus *(530)*
   _____ Concussion *(541)*
   _____ Decerebrate *(550)*
   _____ Decorticate *(550)*

   a. Short period of sleep following a seizure
   b. Farsighted
   c. Incision of the tympanic membrane
   d. Involuntary continual jerking movements of the eyeball
   e. Adduction of arms, flexed on chest with wrists flexed, hands fisted, and feet are in plantar flexion
   f. Edema and inflammation of the optic nerve
   g. Temporary disturbance of the brain usually followed by a period of unconsciousness
   h. Removal of the eye
   i. Rigid extension and pronation of the arms and legs
   j. Crossed eyes

2. An acute infection of the external ear canal is called _____ _____ or _____ _____. *(525)*

3. True or false? *(525-526)*

   a. When a child has otitis externa, the tympanic membrane is erythematous. _____

   b. Prolonged exposure to moisture is a precipitating factor for otitis externa. _____

   c. Otitis media frequently occurs after a child has an upper respiratory infection. _____

4. Explain why infants are more prone to ear infections than older children. *(525)*_____
   _____
   _____
   _____

5. List the main symptoms of otitis media. *(526)* _____
   _____
   _____

6. List two possible complications of recurrent episodes of otitis media. *(527)*

   a. _____

   b. _____

7. Describe the treatment of otitis media. *(527)* _____

   _____

   _____

8. What teaching should be done when antibiotics are prescribed for children with acute otitis media? *(527, Nursing Tip)*

   _____

   _____

   _____

9. Complete bilateral deafness is usually discovered during _____, but partial deafness may be unrecognized until _____. *(528)*

10. Identify assessment findings that might indicate a hearing problem. *(528)*

    a. Infant

       i. _____

       ii. _____

       iii. _____

    b. Older child

       i. _____

       ii. _____

       iii. _____

11. Describe three or more strategies the nurse can use when caring for a hospitalized school-age child who has a hearing impairment. *(528)*

    a. _____

    b. _____

    c. _____

12. Identify one strategy to relieve a child's discomfort resulting from a change in altitude or barometric pressure during airplane descent. *(529)*

    _____

    _____

13. During a visual assessment, the nurse should observe the eyes for: *(530)*

    a. _____

    b. _____

14. Visual acuity can be tested by _____ to _____ years of age. *(530)*

15. For amblyopia, describe the following. *(530)*

    a. Goal of treatment: _____

    _____

    b. Treatment: _____

    _____

16. Why might a child be embarrassed when being treated for amblyopia? *(530, Nursing Tip)* _____

    _____

    _____

    _____

17. Untreated strabismus can result in _____ of one eye. *(531)*

18. Describe the procedure for wiping secretions from the eye in the child with conjunctivitis. *(532)*

    _____

    _____

19. How would the nurse position a child who has a hyphema? *(532)* _____

    _____

20. List the clinical manifestations of retinoblastoma. *(533)* _____

    _____

21. Neural tube development occurs about the _____ to _____ week of fetal life. *(533)*

22. What medication, when used during a viral illness, has been linked to Reye's syndrome? *(533)*

    _____

23. Which two immunizations are recommended to prevent sepsis for all children between 2 months and 4 years of age? *(536)*

    a. _____

    b. _____

24. List five signs and symptoms of meningitis. *(536, Safety Alert)*

    a. _____

    b. _____

    c. _____

    d. _____

    e. _____

25. List treatment measures for the child with meningitis. *(537)*

    a. _____

    b. _____

    c. _____

    d. _____

26. List two measures the nurse should take to decrease stimuli when caring for a child with meningitis. *(537)*

    a. _____

    b. _____

27. The majority of brain tumors in children are located in the _____
    _____. *(538)*

28. The manifestations of a brain tumor are directly related to the _____ and
    _____ of the tumor. *(538)*

29. Most brain tumors create increased _____ _____,
    producing symptoms such as _____, _____,
    _____, and _____. *(538)*

30. Preoperative care of a child with a brain tumor should address what body image issue? *(538)*

    _____

31. Febrile seizures occur in response to a(n) _____. *(539)*

32. What should the nurse observe and record after a seizure? *(539)*

    a. _____

    b. _____

    c. _____

    d. _____

    e. _____

    f. _____

    g. _____

33. Match each classification of seizure with its description (a–d). *(540, Table 23-2)*

    _____ Generalized tonic-clonic seizure
    _____ Absence seizure
    _____ Partial seizure
    _____ Myoclonic seizure

    a. Temporary loss of awareness
    b. Can be manifested by motor activities, sensory signs, or psychomotor activity
    c. Repetitive muscle contractions
    d. Has three phases: aura, seizure, and postictal period

34. What is the term meaning a prolonged seizure that does not respond to treatment for 30 minutes or more? *(541)*

    _____

35. One of the most common causes of status epilepticus is _____
    _____.
    (541)

36. List four or more common causes of cerebral palsy. *(543)*

    a. _____

    b. _____

    c. _____

    d. _____

37. List three clinical manifestations that might indicate a child has cerebral palsy. *(543-544)*

    a. _____

    b. _____

    c. _____

38. List three precautions that should be taken when the nurse is feeding a toddler with cerebral palsy. *(545; Skill 23-1)*

    a. _____

    b. _____

    c. _____

39. Nurses can contribute to the prevention of intellectual impairment by promoting: *(548)*

    a. _____

    b. _____

    c. _____

    d. _____

40. Identify the following illustrations as *decorticate* or *decerebrate* posturing and name the most likely area of injury to the brain for each. *(550, Fig. 23-13)*

a. _____

_____

b. _____

_____

41. The four components of a neurologic check are: *(550, Box 23-6, Table 23-6, Safety Alert)*

a. _____

b. _____

c. _____

d. _____

42. List three questions you might ask a 4-year-old child to help determine his or her level of consciousness. *(550; 551, Nursing Care Plan 23-1)*

a. _____

b. _____

c. _____

43. Vital sign changes suggestive of increased intracranial pressure include: *(552)*

a. _____

b. _____

c. _____

44. Priorities for treatment of a child who experienced near-drowning include immediate treatment of _____, _____, and _____. *(553)*

REVIEW QUESTIONS

1. What information would the nurse give to parents of a young child following surgical insertion of a pressure equalization tube during myringotomy after eardrum rupture? *(527)*
    1. The tube may fall out spontaneously within 6 to 12 months.
    2. Avoid getting water in the child's ears.
    3. Position the child on his back for sleep.
    4. Use cotton swabs to clean the ears.

2. Early signs of Reye's syndrome include: *(533)*
    1. diarrhea and headache.
    2. vomiting and lethargy.
    3. nausea and malaise.
    4. hyperactivity and vomiting.

3. When taking the history of a child with encephalitis, it is important to note recent: *(537)*
    1. cat scratches.
    2. exposure to poison ivy.
    3. respiratory infection.
    4. drug therapy.

4. Which factor is most likely to trigger seizures in a child with epilepsy? *(543; Safety Alert)*
    1. High-fat diet
    2. Hypothermia
    3. Sensitivity to light
    4. Loud noises

5. The nurse recognizes which of the following as symptoms of meningitis? *(536)*
    1. Intense thirst and stiff neck
    2. Hyperactivity and vomiting
    3. Irritability and fever
    4. Loss of vision and malaise

6. A 7-month-old child had a febrile seizure. Which statement would the nurse give to the infant's parents? "Febrile seizures: *(539)*
    1. rarely occur before an infant's first birthday."
    2. indicate a permanent, underlying neurologic problem."
    3. are usually controlled with phenobarbital."
    4. rarely develop into epilepsy."

7. The nurse monitors fluid intake and output in children with a head injury in order to: *(552)*
    1. prevent renal damage.
    2. control cerebral edema.
    3. prevent aspiration.
    4. decrease headaches.

8. Nursing care for a child following a generalized tonic-clonic seizure would include: *(540, Table 23-2)*
    1. attempting to hold the tongue.
    2. administering oxygen.
    3. restraining extremities.
    4. turning on his or her side.

9. The nurse teaching parents about adverse effects of phenytoin (Dilantin) would explain this medication can cause: *(541, 542, Fig. 2-10, Table 23-3)*
   1. drowsiness.
   2. gum overgrowth.
   3. blurred vision.
   4. liver toxicity.

10. Which nursing action is appropriate when caring for a hospitalized child who is hearing-impaired? *(528)*
    1. Speak in a loud, clear tone.
    2. Stand close to the child and speak slowly.
    3. Speak at eye level with the child.
    4. Speak in an exaggerated tone.

11. An infant brought to the emergency department with a high fever, irritability, and a high-pitched cry would immediately be evaluated for: *(536)*
    1. retinoblastoma.
    2. Reye's syndrome.
    3. neuroblastoma.
    4. meningitis.

12. An appropriate nursing intervention for an infant with bacterial meningitis is to: *(537)*
    1. restrain the infant when awake.
    2. position the infant on the right side.
    3. keep the room quiet and indirectly lit.
    4. place in isolation until discharged.

13. Which question will elicit the best information to determine a plan of care during hospitalization for a 5-year-old child who has intellectual impairment? *(548)*
    1. "Can the child dress herself?'
    2. "Is she toilet trained?"
    3. "What is her favorite breakfast food?"
    4. "What is her bedtime routine?"

14. What is the priority for the care of a child with decreased level of consciousness resulting from a head injury? *(554, Nursing Care Plan 23-1)*
    1. Maintain a patent airway.
    2. Prevent skin breakdown.
    3. Monitor fluid balance.
    4. Perform passive range-of-motion exercises.

15. What is an appropriate nursing intervention for feeding a child with spastic-type cerebral palsy? *(545, Skill 23-1)*
    1. Touch the tip of the tongue with the spoon.
    2. Stroke downward under the chin area.
    3. Feed with a rubber-coated spoon.
    4. Tilt the head backward 30 degrees.

CROSSWORD PUZZLE

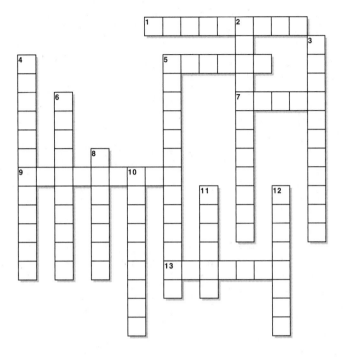

Across

1. Involuntary, purposeless movements *(544)*
5. A movement characterized by an alternating contraction and relaxation of muscles *(539)*
7. A movement characterized by muscle contraction *(539)*
9. A reduction or loss of vision in a child who strongly favors one eye *(530)*
13. Occurrence of sudden, intermittent episodes of altered consciousness, lasting seconds to minutes *(539)*

Down

2. Involuntary arching of the back due to muscle contraction *(536, Fig. 23-8)*
3. Removal of the eye as the standard treatment for retinoblastoma *(533)*
4. Inflammation of the brain *(537)*
5. A group of nonprogressive disorders that affects the motor centers of the brain *(543)*
6. A condition where there is a lack of coordination between the eye muscles that direct movement of the eye *(530)*
8. The presence of blood in the anterior chamber of the eye *(532)*
10. Short period of time following a seizure, usually used to describe a sluggish or sleepy recovery time *(541)*
11. Systemic response caused by bacteria in the bloodstream *(535)*
12. A reading disability that involves a defect in the cortex of the brain that processes graphic symbols *(530)*

CASE STUDIES

1. Jack, age 6 months, is admitted to the hospital with meningitis. He is placed in isolation, an IV is started, and he is on seizure precautions.
   a. How would Jack be positioned for a lumbar puncture?
   b. What changes in Jack's spinal fluid would confirm a diagnosis of meningitis?
   c. State at least six nursing interventions for Jack.

2. Two-year-old Taylor has chronic otitis media with effusion. Audiometric testing shows a mild hearing loss. He is scheduled for a myringotomy with insertion of tympanostomy ventilating tubes (pressure equalizers [PEs]).
   a. How will this surgery improve Taylor's hearing?
   b. What should Taylor's parents know about care of a child with tympanoplasty tubes inserted?

THINKING CRITICALLY

1. You are assigned to care for a 5-year-old child who has a seizure disorder. When you walk into her room, she is watching TV. You are asking the child some questions when her body stiffens. She is unresponsive. Thirty seconds later, her arms and legs begin contracting and relaxing.
   a. What type of seizure is this child experiencing?
   b. What should you do?

APPLYING KNOWLEDGE

1. While in the clinical area, care for a child who is on seizure precautions. What are some of the special procedures you followed?

2. Assist with vision screening in your local school district.

3. Visit your local Easter Seal Society and observe the therapy of children with cerebral palsy. Find out what resources are available for these children.

The Child with a Musculoskeletal Condition

chapter

24

Answer Key: A complete answer key can be found on the Student Evolve website.

LEARNING ACTIVITIES

1. Match the terms in the left column with their definitions on the right (a–h).

    _____ Genu varum *(557)*
    _____ Osteomyelitis *(566)*
    _____ Contusion *(558)*
    _____ Sprain *(558)*
    _____ Strain *(558)*
    _____ Genu valgum *(557)*
    _____ Osteosarcoma *(568)*
    _____ Torticollis *(569)*

    a. Limited neck motion due to shortening of the sternocleidomastoid muscle
    b. Bow-legged or knees turned outward
    c. Knock-kneed or knees turned inward
    d. Tearing of subcutaneous tissue that results in hemorrhage, edema, and pain
    e. A microscopic tear to a muscle or tendon
    f. Infection of the bone
    g. Bone tumor
    h. Ligament that is torn or stretched away from the bone

2. Assessment of the musculoskeletal system in children who can walk includes: *(557)*

    a. _____

    b. _____

    c. _____

    d. _____

3. It is normal for toddlers to have a(n) _____ gait. *(557)*

4. How would the nurse test the strength of a child's extremities? *(558)* _____

    _____

5. True or false? *(557)*

    a. A newborn's feet may turn inward or outward. _____

    b. Children who do not walk independently by 12 months of age should be evaluated for a musculoskeletal problem. _____

    c. Young children may appear "bow-legged" until 5 years of age. _____

    d. A neurologic assessment is part of a comprehensive musculoskeletal assessment. _____

6. List three types of traction used for children. *(558)*

    a. _____

    b. _____

    c. _____

7. Identify three or more differences in the skeletal system of a child as compared to an adult. *(557, Fig. 24-1)*

    a. _____

    b. _____

    c. _____

8. The major signs of a muscle sprain are _____,
    _____, and _____. *(558)*

9. Describe the treatment of a soft tissue injury. *(559, Memory Jogger)* _____

    _____

    _____

    _____

    _____

10. Match the types of fractures in the left column with their definitions on the right (a–d). *(559-560, Safety Alert)*

    _____ Simple   a. Bone is broken but the skin over the area is not broken
    _____ Compound   b. Caused by forceful twisting motion
    _____ Greenstick   c. Open fracture in which the wound in the skin leads to the broken bone
    _____ Spiral   d. Incomplete fracture

11. Bryant's traction is used for treating fractures of the femur in children younger than _____ years of age or less than _____ to _____ pounds. *(560, Fig. 24-3)*

12. You are performing a neurovascular assessment on an infant or child being treated with traction, casting, or Ace bandages. Describe the six findings on the neurovascular assessment that should be reported immediately to the nurse in charge. *(562-563; Skill 24-1; Figure 24-9)*

    a. _____

    b. _____

    c. _____

    d. _____

    e. _____

    f. _____

13. What is Volkmann's ischemia? *(562)* _____

_____

14. Explain split Russell traction. *(560, Fig. 24-4; 561, Nursing Tip; Safety Alert)* _____

_____

_____

_____

_____

_____

15. How is nursing care for a child in skeletal traction different from that for a child in skin traction? *(561)*

_____

_____

16. Complete the following traction-related statements. *(563, Nursing Tip)*

    a. Weights are hanging _____.

    b. Weights are out of reach of _____.

    c. Ropes are on the _____.

    d. Knots are not resting against _____.

    e. Bed linens are not on _____.

    f. _____ is in place.

    g. Apparatus does not touch the _____ of the _____.

17. A priority nursing responsibility in the care of a child with a cast or in traction is _____
_____. *(563)*

18. Pain at the trauma site that is not relieved by analgesics may be a sign of _____
_____. *(563)*

19. A child is receiving intravenous antibiotics for treatment of osteomyelitis. What is a nursing responsibility related to this treatment? *(567)*

_____

20. The most common type of muscular dystrophy is _____. *(567)*

21. List three signs that suggest a child has muscular dystrophy. *(567)*

    a. _____

    b. _____

    c. _____

22. List two or more clinical manifestations of slipped femoral capital epiphysis. *(567-568)*

    a. _____

    b. _____

23. What information should the nurse expect the physician to give parents about the prognosis of Legg-Calvé-Perthes disease in their child? *(568)*

    _____

    _____

    _____

    _____

24. A diagnosis of osteosarcoma is confirmed through a(n) _____. *(568)*

25. What are the goals of care for juvenile idiopathic arthritis (JIR)? *(569)*

    a. _____

    b. _____

    c. _____

    d. _____

    e. _____

26. The two types of scoliosis and the cause for each are: *(570)*

    a. _____

    b. _____

27. The Milwaukee brace must be worn _____ hours a day. *(570, Fig. 24-12)*

28. Screening for scoliosis should be done before _____. *(570)*

29. What does a screening examination for scoliosis involve? *(571)* _____

    _____

    _____

    _____

    _____

30. A child with scoliosis who needs a spinal fusion has special needs related to immobilization. Identify two nursing interventions to prevent gastrointestinal complications from immobility in the postoperative period. *(571)*

    a. _____

    b. _____

31. A parent asks you for guidelines to help prevent injuries in a child who is in competitive sports. List four guidelines. *(571)*

    a. _____

    b. _____

    c. _____

    d. _____

32. What are shin splints? *(572, Table 24-1)* _____

    _____

    _____

33. Describe what the nurse should do if child abuse is suspected. *(573)*

    _____

    _____

    _____

34. What guideline for documentation should the nurse follow when caring for a child who has been abused? *(575, Fig 24-14)*

    _____

    _____

REVIEW QUESTIONS

1. One of the most common causes of death in a child with muscular dystrophy is: *(567)*
   1. renal failure.
   2. osteomyelitis.
   3. cardiac failure.
   4. liver disease.

2. Which type of traction would the nurse expect to be used for a 20-month-old child who has a fractured femur? *(560)*
   1. Buck's extension
   2. Bryant's
   3. Russell's
   4. Ninety-ninety

3. The nurse is aware that a fracture involving the epiphyseal plate in a long bone can result in: *(557, Fig. 24-1)*
   1. reduced red blood cell production.
   2. excessive calcium storage.
   3. impaired bone growth.
   4. delayed bone healing.

4. When a child is referred to a physician after scoliosis screening, the plan is to defer treatment and watch the child. The nurse determines that the child's curvature must be less than: *(570)*
    1. 10 degrees.
    2. 20 degrees.
    3. 30 degrees.
    4. 40 degrees.

5. Which is an expected assessment finding in a child with suspected scoliosis? *(570)*
    1. Prominent clavicle
    2. Expiratory wheeze
    3. Asymmetry of the shoulders
    4. Delayed breast development

6. Which disease is usually inherited as a sex-linked disorder? *(567)*
    1. Legg-Calvé-Perthes disease
    2. Scoliosis
    3. Juvenile idiopathic arthritis
    4. Duchenne's muscular dystrophy

7. The nurse is reinforcing the physician's explanation of treatment for Legg-Calvé-Perthes disease. What information would the nurse review with parents? *(568)*
    1. Buck's extension traction
    2. Muscle strengthening with weights
    3. Surgery to stabilize the joint
    4. Ambulation-abduction casts or braces

8. The nurse completed a neurovascular check on a child in Russell's traction for a fractured femur. Which finding should be reported to the charge nurse? *(565, Nursing Care Plan 24-1, Skill 24-1)*
    1. Foot is warm to the touch.
    2. Can wiggle toes.
    3. Toes feel tingly.
    4. Capillary refill of toes < 3 seconds.

9. The treatment of osteomyelitis includes the use of: *(567)*
    1. steroids.
    2. antibiotics.
    3. traction.
    4. hydrotherapy.

10. The development of uveitis is an autoimmune complication of: *(569)*
    1. Legg-Calvé-Perthes disease.
    2. osteomyelitis.
    3. juvenile rheumatoid arthritis.
    4. torticollis.

11. An appropriate nursing action when caring for a child in Bryant's traction is to: *(560, 562, Fig. 24-3, Nursing Tip, Safety Alert)*
    1. remove the weights when bathing.
    2. support the weights when the bed is moved.
    3. position the child so the buttocks touch the bed.
    4. position the child's legs at right angles to the body.

12. Which is a priority nursing diagnosis for an adolescent treated for osteosarcoma? *(568)*
    1. Risk for infection
    2. Posttrauma syndrome
    3. Disturbed body image
    4. Risk for trauma

13. A toddler has been walking independently for one month. Observation of a toddler's gait reveals the child's feet are wide apart and the gait is unsteady. How would the nurse interpret this finding? *(557)*
    1. The child appears to have genu varum.
    2. Orthotic devices in the shoes will improve the gait.
    3. A comprehensive neurologic assessment is indicated.
    4. This is a normal gait for a child in the toddler age group.

14. The mother of an infant born with congenital torticollis tells the nurse she is concerned that her child will always have limited neck motion. What is the best nursing response to the mother's concern? *(570)*
    1. "Your child will always need to wear a neck brace."
    2. "Surgery is the treatment of choice to correct the problem."
    3. "The condition will most likely resolve by 2–6 months."
    4. "There is nothing you can do to improve the condition."

15. A 3-year-old is being removed from the home of an abusive parent. The child is crying and a co-worker wonders if this could be a sign that the child was not abused. The nurse understands that the child: *(575)*
    1. would not be crying if he or she had been abused in the home.
    2. will mourn the loss of family, even if there was abuse.
    3. is seeking attention from any available adult.
    4. doesn't really understand what is happening.

16. Which statement by a mother might indicate future problems related to the care of a newborn infant? *(572, Health Promotion Box)*
    1. "I am happy that my mother will be here for a few weeks. I will have time to recuperate and adjust to my larger family."
    2. "May I call you with questions? This is my first child and although I feel prepared, I am feeling frightened by the responsibility."
    3. "The baby cries all the time. She doesn't seem to like me. I didn't think it would be like this. Sometimes I think she is just trying to irritate me."
    4. "Our baby has colic. We are taking turns rocking her and getting up with her at night. When will we get a full night of sleep?"

17. What would be the priority nursing intervention when a nurse is caring for a child wearing an Ace bandage for a sprained ankle? *(563, Skill 24-1, Table 24-1)*
    1. Ensure the ankle is elevated on a pillow.
    2. Perform a neurovascular assessment.
    3. Apply a fresh ice pack to the sprained ankle.
    4. Determine when the child received analgesia.

CASE STUDY

1. Olivia, 20 months old, is admitted to the hospital with a fractured femur. She is placed in Bryant's traction.
   a. Olivia's mother asks why this particular type of traction is used. How should the nurse reply?
   b. What particular areas of Olivia's body would be assessed? Provide rationales.
   c. What are some diversional activities the nurse could plan for the child? Base the plan on knowledge of growth and development and Olivia's necessary traction limits. See Chapter 15 for ideas.

THINKING CRITICALLY

1. Nurses who care for abused children may have negative feelings toward the adult who abused the child. Examine your thoughts on this issue. Consider how supporting the adult will ultimately help the child.

2. Identify the steps required in your school system to arrange for school tutoring of a fourth-grade child who is expected to be hospitalized with traction for 4 or more weeks with a femur fracture suffered in a motor vehicle accident. If possible, interview a teacher about adaptations he or she must often make in teaching to enhance learning in children with health problems that confine them to acute care or rehabilitation facilities.

APPLYING KNOWLEDGE

1. While in the clinical area, care for a child in traction. Practice a neurovascular assessment on this child or a classmate.

2. Screen a 10-year-old girl (or middle-school girl) for scoliosis.

3. Give skin care to a child (or adult) with skeletal traction.

4. Plan a presentation on sports injury prevention for school-age children with your classmates.

5. Label the following bones on the figure below. Check your answers with an anatomy textbook. Enlarge this figure for labeling if you wish.

    a. Femur
    b. Tibia
    c. Fibula
    d. Ulna
    e. Radius
    f. Coccyx
    g. Clavicle
    h. Humerus

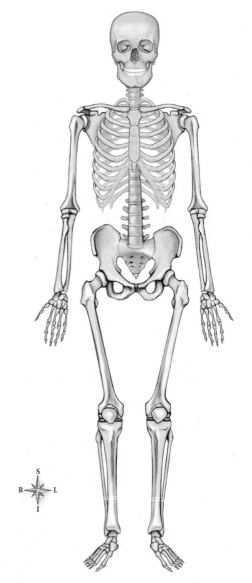

The Child with a Respiratory Disorder

Answer Key: A complete answer key can be found on the Student Evolve website.

LEARNING ACTIVITIES

1. Match the terms in the left column with their definitions on the right (a–g).

   _____ Allergic salute *(588, Fig. 25-4)*
   _____ Alveoli *(584, Fig 25-1, Table 25-1)*
   _____ Dysphagia *(580)*
   _____ Orthopnea *(581)*
   _____ Status asthmaticus *(595)*
   _____ Stridor *(581, Fig. 25-2)*
   _____ Surfactant *(577)*

   a. Combination of lecithin and sphingomyelin
   b. Harsh, high-pitched sound on inspiration
   c. Asthma attack that is not responsive to drugs
   d. Rubbing nose in response to nasal discharge
   e. Air sacs surrounded by capillaries for gas exchange
   f. Requiring upright positioning to breathe
   g. Difficult swallowing

2. The common cold is also known as _____ _____. *(578, Medication Safety Alert, Nursing Tip)*

3. List five measures that can relieve symptoms of the common cold. *(579, Nursing Tip)*

   a. _____

   b. _____

   c. _____

   d. _____

   e. _____

4. a. The child with a strep throat is no longer infectious when _____
   _____. *(580)*

   b. What complications can arise when strep throat is not treated promptly? *(580)*

   _____

   _____

5. What is the treatment for sinusitis? *(581)* _____

6. Define the term *croup*. (581) _____

_____

_____

_____

7. Describe the clinical course of laryngotracheobronchitis. (581)_____

_____

_____

_____

_____

8. What advice would you give a parent about home care of a child with croup? (582) _____

_____

_____

_____

_____

9. If epiglottitis is suspected, what nursing responsibility must be instituted? (582, *Safety Alert*)

_____

10. If subglottic edema occurs, it can result in _____ because the area
    below the glottis is made up of _____ that cannot _____. (581)

11. List the common signs and symptoms of bronchiolitis. (583)

    a. _____

    b. _____

    c. _____

    d. _____

    e. _____

12. What position facilitates breathing for the infant with bronchiolitis? (583)_____

_____

13. Respiratory syncytial virus (RSV) is spread by direct contact with _____
    _____. (583)

14. RSV can survive for more than _____ hours on countertops, tissues, and soap. (583)

15. The priority nursing diagnosis for an infant hospitalized with RSV infection is _____
    _____. (584)

16. List four of the possible signs of respiratory distress. *(581; Figure 25-2)*

    a. _____

    b. _____

    c. _____

    d. _____

17. Describe four or more of the common signs and symptoms of pneumonia. *(585)*

    a. _____

    b. _____

    c. _____

    d. _____

18. Home care for a child with pneumonia involves: *(585)*

    a. _____

    b. _____

    c. _____

19. The removal of the tonsils and adenoids should wait until the child is at least _____ years of age. *(586)*

20. What signs and symptoms are indicative of bleeding in the postoperative tonsillectomy patient? *(588)*

    a. _____

    b. _____

    c. _____

    d. _____

21. What are the characteristic signs of allergic rhinitis? *(588, Fig. 25-4)* _____

    _____

22. Describe the pathologic changes that take place in asthma. *(589)*_____

    _____

    _____

    _____

    _____

    _____

23. List five or more signs and symptoms of an acute asthma episode. *(590, Safety Alert)*

    a. _____

    b. _____

    c. _____

    d. _____

    e. _____

24. Describe nursing considerations when administering albuterol to a child with asthma. *(591, Table 25-2)*

    _____

    _____

    _____

    _____

25. What should the nurse teach the family of a child with asthma about administering cromolyn sodium daily to inhibit response to allergens and exercise-induced asthma? *(591, Table 25-2)*

    _____

    _____

    _____

    _____

26. What should the nurse teach the family of a child with asthma about controlling allergens in the child's bedroom? *(591)*

    _____

    _____

    _____

    _____

27. Why should a child with asthma use a spacer with a metered-dose inhaler? *(593)* _____

    _____

28. Cystic fibrosis is a(n) _____ _____ trait caused by a defect in _____. *(595)*

29. Describe how cystic fibrosis affects the child's respiratory system. *(596, Fig. 25-9)* _____

    _____

    _____

    _____

    _____

30. Describe the stools of a child with cystic fibrosis. *(596)* _____

_____

31. What physiologic changes take place in the pancreas of a child with cystic fibrosis? *(597)* _____

_____

_____

_____

32. A(n) _____ _____ is the test of choice for diagnosing cystic fibrosis. *(597)*

33. Describe three ways respiratory complications can be decreased in patients with cystic fibrosis. *(596; 597, Nursing Care Plan 25-1; 600-601, Figure 25-11)*

    a. _____

    _____

    b. _____

    _____

    c. _____

    _____

34. Specific parent teaching for administration of an oral pancreatic agent to a child with cystic fibrosis should include: *(598, 599)*

    _____

    _____

    _____

    _____

    _____

35. Children with cystic fibrosis should receive which vitamin and mineral supplements? *(599)*

    _____

    _____

36. What is the best way to prevent bronchopulmonary dysplasia? *(602, Safety Alert)* _____

    _____

37. The nurse teaches parents to place infants in the _____ position for sleep. This measure reduces the risk of _____. *(602; 603, Safety Alert)*

REVIEW QUESTIONS

1. An appropriate intervention for a child with bronchiolitis is: *(583)*
    1. isolation.
    2. increased fluids.
    3. supine for sleeping.
    4. dry environment.

2. What is the best liquid for the nurse to give to a child who has had a tonsillectomy? *(588, 588, Nursing Tips)*
    1. Apple juice
    2. Milk
    3. Sweet or diet colas
    4. Fresh-squeezed lemonade

3. The nurse determines a parent understands diet teaching for a child with cystic fibrosis when she states the child should eat which type of diet? *(599)*
    1. High calorie, high protein, no salt supplement
    2. High calorie, with salt supplement
    3. Low calorie, high protein, low salt
    4. Low calorie, low protein, with salt supplement

4. The nurse places a child with croup in an environment of high humidity for which effect? *(582)*
    1. Decrease the possibility of dehydration
    2. Decrease risk of spreading the infection
    3. Decrease mucosal swelling
    4. Decrease risk of vomiting and aspiration

5. An appropriate nursing action when a child is suspected of having epiglottitis is to: *(582)*
    1. avoid examination of the pharynx.
    2. collect a throat culture.
    3. place the child on the right side.
    4. institute isolation precautions.

6. The nurse observes a child who had a tonsillectomy a few hours earlier is swallowing frequently. What is the appropriate action for the nurse to take? *(588, 588, Nursing Tips)*
    1. Offer the child cold milk.
    2. Reposition the child to supine.
    3. Instruct the child to cough or clear the throat.
    4. Notify the physician.

7. What information would be included in a teaching plan for a child with asthma? *(593, 594)*
    1. Avoid exercise and sports activities.
    2. Keep house humidity above 50%.
    3. Identify early signs of an asthma attack.
    4. Decrease the amount of liquids taken after 6:00 PM.

8. The nurse would expect the parent of an infant with croup to describe the infant's cough as: *(581)*
    1. dry.
    2. barking.
    3. productive.
    4. quiet.

9. Which instruction is most helpful for administering albuterol to a child with asthma? *(591, Table 25-2)*
   1. Take 30-60 minutes before exercise.
   2. Child should hold breath 5-10 seconds after inhaling or use a spacer.
   3. Give with food to reduce gastric irritation.
   4. Administer in early AM when normal hormones peak.

10. A 3-year-old boy was seen in the clinic by the pediatrician and diagnosed with pneumonia. Amoxicillin for 10 days was prescribed, with a follow-up visit in 2 weeks. Choose the priority parent teaching. *(585-586; Pictorial Pathway 12-1)*
    1. Avoid giving cough medication at naptime or bedtime.
    2. Importance of taking all of the prescribed amoxicillin.
    3. Wrap snuggly in blankets till fever breaks.
    4. Room-temperature, fizzy soft drinks enhance amoxicillin absorption.

CASE STUDIES

1. Six-year-old Jasmine is admitted to the hospital with a diagnosis of asthma. She is restless, has difficulty breathing, and is wheezing. She has numerous allergies.
   a. Jasmine's dad relates that she has been taking allergy shots and that the family has removed many of the objects she is allergic to from their home. Explain each of these methods of allergy treatment.
   b. What position should Jasmine assume to decrease respiratory distress?
   c. The physician wants Jasmine to have increased fluid intake. What liquids should be encouraged and which should be avoided?
   d. Jasmine wants to participate in the beginners' swim team at school. What should the nurse tell her about asthma and exercise?
   e. Explain to Jasmine how to use a metered-dose inhaler for her medication.

2. Alicia, an 8-year-old child, is admitted to the hospital with respiratory problems related to cystic fibrosis. She has a history of chronic pulmonary and sinus problems.
   a. Alicia takes an oral pancreatic enzyme. When should she take this medication?
   b. Alicia has extensive lung disease. What measures would improve respiration?
   c. What type of diet would be ordered for Alicia?
   d. Alicia's appetite has markedly decreased. What can be done to increase her intake?

THINKING CRITICALLY

1. Plan for the discharge of a child newly diagnosed with cystic fibrosis. Include diet, medication, respiratory care, and psychological care of the child and the parents.

2. Look up the latest statistics for preterm births in the United States (www.cdc.gov/nchs/fastats/birthwt.htm).

APPLYING KNOWLEDGE

1. Care for a child in an oxygen tent who has a respiratory disease.

2. Look up infection control policy on isolation for RSV and who is restricted from providing care if the child is receiving ribavirin (Virazole).

3. Admit a child who has asthma to the unit.

4. Teach a child with cystic fibrosis or the parent about respiratory care and diet.

The Child with a Cardiovascular Disorder

Answer Key: A complete answer key can be found on the Student Evolve website.

LEARNING ACTIVITIES

1. Match the terms in the left column with their definitions on the right (a–f).

   _____ Chorea *(614)*
   _____ "Tet" spell *(610, Fig. 26-3)*
   _____ Hemodynamics *(606)*
   _____ Polycythemia *(609)*
   _____ Pulse pressure *(609)*
   _____ Shunt *(606)*

   a. Blood flow through an abnormal opening between two vessels
   b. Difference between highest and lowest blood pressure levels
   c. Paroxysmal hypercyanotic episode
   d. Increased red blood cells
   e. Study of blood circulation
   f. CNS disorder characterized by involuntary, purposeless movements

2. List at least five signs that indicate an infant may have a congenital cardiac problems. *(605)*

   a. _____

   b. _____

   c. _____

   d. _____

   e. _____

3. _____ _____ are the leading cause of death among the congenital anomalies during the first year of life. *(606)*

4. Heart defects can be classified as lesions that: *(606)*

   a. _____

   b. _____

   c. _____

5. Match the types of heart defects on the left with their definitions on the right (a–d).

    _____ Ventricular septal defect *(608)*

    _____ Coarctation of the aorta *(609)*

    _____ Atrial septal defect *(607)*

    _____ Patent ductus arteriosus *(608)*

a. Narrowing of the aortic arch or the descending aorta

b. Opening between the right and left ventricles

c. Failure of the ductus arteriosus to close

d. Opening between left and right atria

6. When a ventricular septal defect is present, higher pressure in the _____ ventricle forces blood back into the _____ ventricle. The defect causes a(n) _____ to _____ shunting of blood. *(608)*

7. a. Why are prophylactic antibiotics given to children with heart disease? *(610)* _____

    _____

    b. When are prophylactic antibiotics likely to be given to a child with a congenital defect? *(611)*

    _____

8. Describe the characteristic murmur associated with patent ductus arteriosus. *(609)* _____

    _____

9. What is the classic sign of coarctation of the aorta? *(609)* _____

    _____

10. Describe the four defects that make up tetralogy of Fallot. *(609)*

    a. _____

    b. _____

    c. _____

    d. _____

11. Explain why polycythemia develops in children with tetralogy of Fallot. *(609)* _____

    _____

    _____

12. How would the nurse position an infant experiencing a paroxysmal hypercyanotic episode? *(610)*

    _____

13. List four or more signs and symptoms of congestive heart failure. *(611; 612, Safety Alert)*

    a. _____

    b. _____

    c. _____

    d. _____

14. Respirations over _____ breaths/minute in a newborn at rest indicate distress. *(612)*

15. What two tips can help the parents of a child with congenital heart disease conserve the child's energy? *(611)*

    a. _____

    _____

    b. _____

    _____

16. Offer two vacation tips to the parents of a child with polycythemia. *(611)*

    a. _____

    _____

    b. _____

    _____

17. Children receiving diuretics must have their serum _____ monitored closely. *(613)*

18. List four foods high in potassium. *(613)*

    a. _____

    b. _____

    c. _____

    d. _____

19. List five signs and symptoms of digitalis toxicity. *(612)*

    a. _____

    b. _____

    c. _____

    d. _____

    e. _____

20. What are the classic signs and symptoms of rheumatic fever? *(613)*

    a. _____

    b. _____

    c. _____

    d. _____

21. Rheumatic fever can be avoided by identification of _____ infections and treatment with _____. *(613)*

22. What advice would you give an adolescent who shows a consistently high blood pressure reading? *(616, Nursing Tip, Health Promotion boxes)*

_____

_____

23. Kawasaki's disease causes _____ of the vessels in the cardiovascular system, which can result in _____. *(617)*

24. Name three medications that may be used in the treatment of Kawasaki's disease. *(618)*

a. _____

b. _____

c. _____

REVIEW QUESTIONS

1. What is the most common congenital heart defect occurring in children? *(608)*
   1. Ventricular septal defect
   2. Coarctation of the aorta
   3. Atrial septal defect
   4. Patent ductus arteriosus

2. What is the best method of feeding an infant in congestive heart failure from a large ventricular septal defect? *(612)*
   1. Space feedings at least every 3–4 hours.
   2. Give frequent, large feedings.
   3. Feed intravenously.
   4. Feed smaller amounts more frequently.

3. Digoxin (Lanoxin) is withheld if the pulse of a newborn is lower than _____ bpm. *(612)*
   1. 120
   2. 110
   3. 100
   4. 90

4. When an infant is receiving digoxin (Lanoxin), the nurse would be alert to which finding as a sign of toxicity? *(612)*
   1. Fluid retention
   2. Diarrhea
   3. Nausea and vomiting
   4. Weight loss

5. A nurse's responsibility when a child is receiving diuretics is to: *(613)*
   1. withhold fluids.
   2. monitor serum electrolyte levels.
   3. place on seizure precautions.
   4. check the dosage with another nurse before administering.

6. Hypertension is identified in a 10-year-old child during routine screening. Which plan of care can the nurse expect to see implemented initially? *(616, Health Promotion box)*
   1. The child is started on a diuretic.
   2. Beta-adrenergic blockers are prescribed.
   3. An exercise and diet program is developed.
   4. A blood pressure measurement is scheduled in 4 weeks.

7. An infant with tetralogy of Fallot becomes hypercyanotic. The nurse would place the infant in the _____ position. *(610)*
   1. high Fowler's
   2. Trendelenburg
   3. side-lying
   4. knee-chest

8. An infant with congestive heart failure would most likely experience: *(612)*
   1. excess or rapid weight gain.
   2. difficulty feeding.
   3. bradypnea.
   4. erythema.

9. A congenital heart defect that results in decreased pulmonary blood flow is: *(609)*
   1. tetralogy of Fallot.
   2. atrial septal defect.
   3. ventricular septal defect.
   4. patent ductus arteriosus.

10. The nurse measuring an infant's blood pressure finds it is higher in the arms than the legs. The finding is associated with which congenital heart defect? *(619)*
    1. Tetralogy of Fallot
    2. Coarctation of the aorta
    3. Patent ductus arteriosus
    4. Hypoplastic left heart syndrome

CROSSWORD PUZZLE

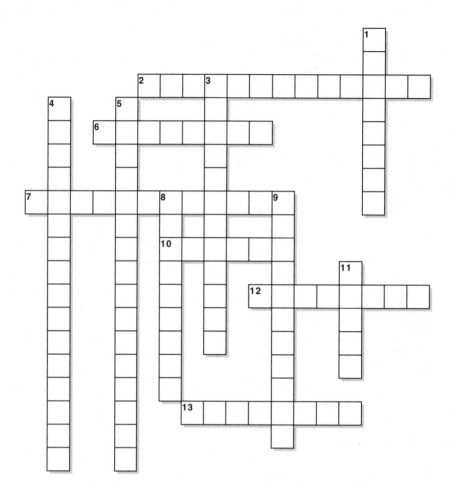

Across

2. Difference between the systolic and diastolic blood pressures (two words) *(609)*
6. Heart disease occurring after birth *(606)*
7. Increased number of red blood cells *(609)*
10. Disorder characterized by involuntary, purposeless movements *(614)*
12. Narrowing of a vessel *(609)*
13. Inflammation of the heart *(614)*

Down

1. Enlargement of fingertips as compensatory response to chronic lack of oxygen *(609; Figure 25-10)*
3. Amount of blood ejected during one heart contraction (two words) *(612)*
4. Prevention of disease by drugs *(615)*
5. Procedure that enables diagnosis of cardiac defects in the fetus *(616)*
8. Higher-than-normal respiratory rate *(612)*
9. Natural or surgical joining of tubular structures *(609)*
11. Major and minor criteria to identify rheumatic fever *(614)*

THINKING CRITICALLY

1. You are caring for a 1-month-old infant with a ventricular septal defect who is in heart failure. When you assessed the infant's apical heart rate before his 8:00 AM dose of Lanoxin, it was 112 bpm. Should you administer the Lanoxin?

2. Develop a teaching plan for 17-year-old adolescent with a serum cholesterol level of 199 mg/dL.

APPLYING KNOWLEDGE

1. Observe a cardiac catheterization in the clinical area.

2. Care for a child with cardiac disease.

3. Care for a child who has had cardiac surgery.

4. With a partner in class, choose foods that you like that can raise the HDL ("good") cholesterol and lower the LDL ("bad") cholesterol.
   a. Can you make a lunch to take to work or school from these foods?
   b. What are the best drinks to have with your lunch?
   c. Have you identified any changes needed in your diet?

5. Participate in a community blood pressure screening when available.

The Child with a Condition of the Blood, Blood-Forming Organs, or Lymphatic System	chapter **27**

Answer Key: A complete answer key can be found on the Student Evolve website.

LEARNING ACTIVITIES

1. Match the terms in the left column with their definitions on the right (a–g).

   _____ Alopecia *(631)*
   _____ Erythrocytes *(621)*
   _____ Hemarthrosis *(628)*
   _____ Leukocytes *(621)*
   _____ Petechiae *(621)*
   _____ Purpura *(621)*
   _____ Thrombocytes *(621)*

   a. Red blood cells (RBCs)
   b. Pinpoint hemorrhagic spots beneath the skin
   c. White blood cells (WBCs)
   d. Platelets
   e. Hemorrhage into a joint cavity
   f. Loss of hair
   g. Large hemorrhagic spots in the skin

2. State the functions of the following blood components. *(621)*

   a. Leukocytes: _____

   b. Erythrocytes: _____

   c. Thrombocytes: _____

3. List the causes of iron-deficiency anemia. *(622; Nursing Care Plan 27-1)*

   a. _____

   b. _____

   c. _____

   d. _____

4. List four food sources with high iron content. *(622; Nursing Care Plan 27-1; Nursing Tip)*

   a. _____

   b. _____

   c. _____

   d. _____

5. List the major signs and symptoms of iron-deficiency anemia. *(622; Nursing Care Plan 27-1)*

   a. _____

   b. _____

   c. _____

   d. _____

6. Full-term infants should be screened for iron-deficiency anemia at _____ and _____ months of age. *(622)*

7. What instructions would you give to a parent about administering an iron supplement to a toddler? *(622)*

   _____

   _____

   _____

8. Describe the stools of a young child receiving an iron supplement. *(622)* _____

   _____

9. What should the nurse tell a parent about formula and milk intake during the first year of life? *(622)*

   _____

   _____

   _____

10. Sickle cell disease is most prevalent in people of _____ or _____ descent. *(623)*

11. List four factors that might trigger a sickle cell crisis. *(624)*

    a. _____

    b. _____

    c. _____

    d. _____

12. Explain the difference between sickle cell trait and sickle cell disease. *(624)* _____

    _____

    _____

    _____

13. The child with sickle cell disease inherits the abnormality from _____ parent(s). *(624)*

14. Name and describe the four types of sickle cell crises. *(625; Table 27-1; Nursing Tip)*

    a. _____

    b. _____

    c. _____

    d. _____

15. a. What is the most common test used to screen for sickle cell disease? *(624)* _____

    b. What test is done if the screening test is positive and why? *(624)* _____

    _____

16. Why is meperidine not recommended for children with sickle cell disease? *(626, Medication Safety Alert)*

    _____

17. Patient-controlled analgesia can be used for the child older than _____ years of age to manage pain caused by sickle cell crisis. *(626)*

18. List two priority goals when caring for a child with sickle cell disease. *(626)*

    a. _____

    b. _____

19. a. The mainstay of treatment for thalassemia major is _____ .

    b. What does this treatment maintain? _____ *(627)*

20. Children with thalassemia major develop _____ as a result of treatment. *(627)*

21. Hemophilia is inherited by the male as a(n) _____ _____ trait. *(628)*

22. Hemophilia A is caused by a deficiency of _____ _____ , while hemophilia B is a(n) _____ _____ deficiency. *(628)*

23. A classic symptom of hemophilia is severe joint pain, which is caused by _____ , also known as hemorrhage into a(n) _____ _____ . *(628)*

24. The principal therapy for hemophilia is to prevent _____ by replacing the missing factor. *(628)*

25. _____ _____ (_____) is a nasal spray that can stop bleeding and may be the treatment of choice for mild cases of hemophilia. *(629; Medication Safety Alert, salicylates contraindicated)*

26. When bleeding occurs from minor trauma in a child with hemophilia, the traditional approach is to use these four steps (RICE): *(628)*

    a. _____

    b. _____

    c. _____

    d. _____

27. Describe the clinical manifestations of idiopathic (immunologic) thrombocytopenic purpura (ITP). *(629; Medication Safety Alert, anti-D antibody observations)*

_____

_____

_____

_____

28. a. The most common form of childhood cancer is _____. *(630)*

    b. This type of cancer results in the uncontrolled growth of _____

    _____. *(630)*

29. Explain the pathologic changes that take place when a child has leukemia. *(630)*_____

_____

_____

_____

_____

_____

30. List at least seven of the possible presenting signs and symptoms of leukemia. *(630)*

    a. _____

    b. _____

    c. _____

    d. _____

    e. _____

    f. _____

    g. _____

31. List the five phases of chemotherapy for leukemia. *(631; Nursing Tip)*

    a. _____

    b. _____

    c. _____

    d. _____

    e. _____

32. List some of the common side effects of chemotherapy. *(630)*

    a. _____

    b. _____

    c. _____

    d. _____

    e. _____

33. Identify three nursing interventions appropriate for a 10-year-old girl who is worried about her body image changes associated with chemotherapy. *(631; Nursing Care Plan 27-2)*

    a. _____

    b. _____

    c. _____

34. List five signs of a transfusion reaction. *(632; 633, Nursing Tip)*

    a. _____

    b. _____

    c. _____

    d. _____

    e. _____

35. If a child showed signs of a transfusion reaction, the nurse's initial action would be to _____ _____. *(632; Nursing Tip)*

36. True or false? *(633)*

    a. Hodgkin's disease is a malignancy of the lymphatic system. _____

    b. The presenting sign of Hodgkin's disease is usually pain in the neck and shoulders. _____

    c. The treatment of Hodgkin's disease involves chemotherapy and radiation therapy. _____

37. Following a splenectomy, the child faces the long-term risk of serious _____. *(627)*

38. Describe the preschooler's response to the death of a sibling. *(638; Health Promotion, 638; Nursing Tip, brothers and sisters; Nursing Care Plan 27-3, 639)*

    _____

    _____

39. The primary fear of dying in children younger than 5 years of age concerns _____ _____. *(637; Health Promotion, 638; Nursing Care Plan 27-3, 639)*

40. Children develop an understanding of death as permanent around age _____ years. *(637; Health Promotion, 638; Nursing Care Plan 27-3, 639)*

REVIEW QUESTIONS

1. By what age do children realize that death is final and permanent? *(637, 638)*
   1. 3 years
   2. 5 years
   3. 7 years
   4. 10 years

2. Iron supplement absorption is increased by taking it with: *(622, Nursing Tip)*
   1. orange juice.
   2. cereal.
   3. milk.
   4. eggs.

3. It is recommended that iron-fortified formula be given to infants through age: *(622)*
   1. 3 months.
   2. 6 months.
   3. 9 months.
   4. 12 months.

4. Which of the following presents the greatest risk to the child with hemophilia? *(629)*
   1. Hematuria
   2. Hemarthrosis
   3. Intracranial bleeding
   4. Iron deficiency anemia

5. Signs and symptoms that might indicate that a child has ITP include: *(629)*
   1. headaches and hematuria.
   2. anemia and purpura.
   3. petechiae and purpura.
   4. hematuria and petechiae.

6. The diagnostic test that confirms a diagnosis of leukemia is a(n): *(629)*
   1. spinal tap.
   2. bone marrow aspiration.
   3. complete blood count.
   4. x-ray of the bones.

7. When caring for a child on steroid therapy, it is important to seek immediate medical attention if the child: *(631-632)*
   1. vomits.
   2. develops a fever.
   3. skips a meal.
   4. loses her hair.

8. Children with Hodgkin's disease usually present with a(n): *(633)*
   1. unexpected sudden weight gain.
   2. painless cervical neck lump.
   3. enlarged abdomen.
   4. high fever.

9. Children with hemophilia should avoid: *(629, Medication Safety Alert)*
   1. swimming.
   2. salicylates.
   3. citrus fruits.
   4. analgesics.

10. Children who carry the sickle cell trait: *(624)*
    1. have a 10% chance of developing the disease.
    2. have a 25% chance of developing the disease.
    3. have a 50% chance of developing the disease.
    4. will not develop any symptoms of the disease.

11. An appropriate nursing intervention for the child admitted to the hospital in sickle cell crisis would be to: *(624, 626)*
    1. apply ice to painful areas.
    2. encourage the child to ambulate.
    3. provide foods high in iron at meals.
    4. monitor the child's response to analgesics.

12. Immediate nursing care of a child with hemophilia who has hemarthrosis includes: *(628, 629)*
    1. application of heat.
    2. active and passive range-of-motion exercises.
    3. immobilization of the area of pain.
    4. withholding factor VIII.

13. The greatest concern of a nurse caring for a child with ITP is: *(629)*
    1. injuries that might initiate bleeding.
    2. a reaction to excess platelets.
    3. noncompliance with aspirin therapy.
    4. development of a secondary bacterial infection.

14. Anxiety can be decreased in both the family and the child who has cancer by: *(632)*
    1. not telling the child that he or she has cancer.
    2. explaining all procedures before they are done.
    3. placing the child with an older child who has the same diagnosis.
    4. discouraging the child and parents from discussing the issue of death.

15. A child with newly diagnosed leukemia does not have all immunizations up to date. Which is an essential step in response to this? *(631)*
    1. Delay treatment till all immunizations have taken effect because a child with leukemia is immunocompromised and prone to serious illness.
    2. Delay active immunizations during chemotherapy.
    3. Administer immunizations on alternating days from chemotherapy.
    4. Give immunizations according to the expected schedule; they do not interfere with treatment.

16. Nursing care of an adolescent with cancer who is refusing to cooperate with treatment should include: *(635; Nursing Care Plan 27-2; 636, Table 27-3)*
    1. allowing the adolescent to make some choices.
    2. asking the parents to make the adolescent cooperate.
    3. restricting visits from friends until the behavior is modified.
    4. withholding the influences of group therapy until the behavior changes.

17. What would be the initial nursing action when a child receiving a transfusion of packed red blood cells complains of chills and back pain? *(632, Nursing Tip)*
    1. Reduce the infusion rate.
    2. Take the child's blood pressure.
    3. Administer Benadryl as ordered.
    4. Discontinue the transfusion.

CROSSWORD PUZZLE

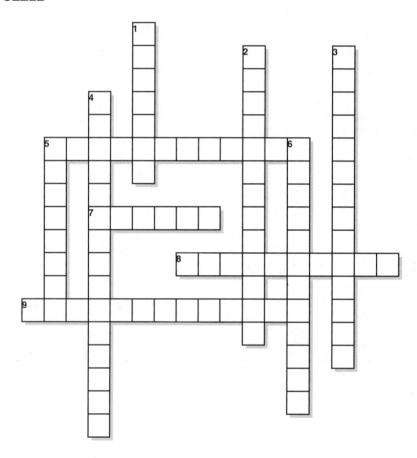

Across

5. Bleeding into a joint space *(628)*
7. A reduction in the size of RBCs or in amount of circulating hemoglobin *(622, Nursing Care Plan 27-1)*
8. A physician who specializes in treating cancer *(630)*
9. Type of sickle cell crisis caused by obstruction of blood flow by abnormally shaped cells *(625, Table 27-1)*

Down

1. Large petechiae *(621)*
2. Deposit of iron into organs and tissues of the body *(626)*
3. Regulates the rate of RBC production *(620)*
4. Enlargement of lymph nodes *(621)*
5. Raised ecchymosis *(629)*
6. Enlargement of the spleen *(621)*

CASE STUDY

1. Lauren, a 5-year-old girl, is hospitalized with acute lymphocytic leukemia (ALL). She is receiving chemotherapy and has been placed in a private room.
    a. What special precautions should be taken with a child who is immune-suppressed?
    b. Lauren develops ulcerations in her mouth. What can the nurse do to relieve discomfort and promote healing of the oral mucosa?
    c. Lauren is to receive a unit of packed red blood cells. For what signs and symptoms of a reaction should the nurse observe and what action would be taken if a reaction occurred?

THINKING CRITICALLY

1. Develop a nursing care plan for a child with sickle cell disease experiencing a vasoocclusive crisis. (*624, 625; Nursing Tip; Table 27-1*)

2. Review the genetic implications of sickle cell disease. Results of hemoglobin electrophoresis show that an infant has sickle cell anemia. The infant's parents desire to have several more children. When both parents have the sickle cell trait, what are the chances that:
    a. a child will have sickle cell anemia?
    b. a child will carry the sickle cell trait?
    c. a child will have neither the disease nor the trait?
    d. Will the child's gender affect whether the child has the disease? Why or why not?

3. Why does a child's gender affect whether he or she is likely to manifest hemophilia?

APPLYING KNOWLEDGE

1. While in the clinical area, care for a child who has cancer and is receiving chemotherapy. Or describe care that you have done for an adult patient who has cancer and is undergoing chemotherapy.

2. While in the clinical area, care for a child who is experiencing sickle cell crisis.

3. Observe a bone marrow aspiration being performed.

The Child with a Gastrointestinal Condition

Answer Key: A complete answer key can be found on the Student Evolve website.

LEARNING ACTIVITIES

1. Match the terms in the left column with their definitions on the right (a–g).

   _____ Homeostasis *(656)*

   _____ Incarceration *(649)*

   _____ Inguinal hernia *(649)*

   _____ Pica *(666)*

   _____ Projectile vomiting *(645)*

   _____ Pyloromyotomy *(645)*

   _____ Plumbism *(666)*

   a. Protrusion of part of the intestine through the umbilical ring
   b. Constriction or irreducibility
   c. Eating nonfood items
   d. Operation to correct pyloric stenosis
   e. State of equilibrium of the body
   f. Vomiting in which the stomach contents are forcibly ejected
   g. Lead poisoning

2. List four or more common tests used to diagnose gastrointestinal disorders. *(643)*

   a. _____

   b. _____

   c. _____

   d. _____

3. The infant with tracheoesophageal fistula will _____ and _____ when the first feeding is given. *(644, Nursing Tip)*

4. Define *pyloric stenosis*. *(645, 646, Clinical Pathway 28-1)* _____

   _____

   _____

5. a. A complication of the vomiting associated with pyloric stenosis is _____.
   (645, 646; Clinical Pathway 28-1)

   b. Describe assessment findings in a newborn who has this complication. *(645, 646)* _____

   _____

   _____

6. Describe the progression of feeding of an infant after postoperative correction of pyloric stenosis. *(645, 646; Clinical Pathway 28-1)*

_____

_____

_____

_____

7. Celiac disease is the leading _____ problem in children. *(647, Safety Alert; Fig. 28-4)*

8. Gluten is found in _____, _____, _____, and _____. *(647)*

9. Stools in the child with celiac disease are _____, _____, and _____. *(647, Safety Alert)*

10. The earliest sign of Hirschsprung's disease is failure to pass meconium stools within _____ to _____ hours after birth. *(648, Fig. 28-5)*

11. Hirschsprung's disease is treated _____. It may be necessary for the infant to have a(n) _____ temporarily. *(648)*

12. Tap-water enemas are never given to children because they can lead to _____ _____ and _____. *(648)*

13. Describe the initial onset of intussusception and infant behaviors. *(648; Fig. 28-6)* _____

_____

_____

_____

14. Treatment of choice for intussusception is reduction through the use of a(n) _____ _____. *(648)*

15. Name and describe the most common congenital malformation of the gastrointestinal tract. *(649)*

_____

16. Surgical repair of a hernia is called a(n) _____. *(650)*

17. The priority goal of nursing care for the infant with gastroenteritis is preventing or correcting _____. *(650, Nursing Tip)*

18. Identify at least three nursing interventions for an infant hospitalized for gastroenteritis. *(650)*

    a. _____

    b. _____

    c. _____

19. Persistent vomiting can result in _____ and _____ _____. *(650)*

20. To prevent aspiration of vomitus after feeding, an infant should be placed in what position? *(651)*

_____

21. What would be included in the nurse's documentation for a child who is vomiting? *(651)*

a. _____

b. _____

c. _____

d. _____

e. _____

f. _____

g. _____

22. Describe *gastroesophageal reflux*. *(651; Nursing Tip)* _____

_____

23. After a feeding, an infant with gastroesophageal reflux should be placed in which position? *(651)*

_____

24. Signs and symptoms of dehydration in the infant with diarrhea include: *(652, 656, Table 28-2; Nursing Care Plan 28-1, 653)*

a. _____

b. _____

c. _____

d. _____

25. A 6-year-old child has mild diarrhea. How would the nurse advise the child's parents about fluid and food intake? *(653; Nursing Care Plan 28-1)*

_____

_____

26. Name three high-fiber foods to recommend to an older child who is experiencing constipation. *(654)*

a. _____

b. _____

c. _____

27. In children under age 2 years, a greater percentage of body water is contained in the _____ compartment. *(654; Safety Alert; Fig,. 28-9)*

28. _____ is the greatest threat to life in isotonic dehydration. *(657)*

29. Failure to thrive (FTT) describes infants and children who _____ _____. *(659)*

30. Kwashiorkor results from a severe deficiency of _____ in the child's diet. *(660)*

31. List four signs of rickets. *(660)*

   a. _____

   b. _____

   c. _____

   d. _____

32. The decreased incidence of rickets in the world is attributed to _____ _____. *(660)*

33. Scurvy results from a deficiency of foods containing _____ in the diet. To prevent scurvy, the nurse would encourage parents to include _____ _____ and _____ _____ _____ in the child's diet. *(660)*

34. True or false? *(660-661)*

   a. With appendicitis, vomiting begins before abdominal pain. _____

   b. Fever is a reliable sign of appendicitis in children. _____

   c. Abdominal pain associated with appendicitis in a child is localized in the right lower quadrant. _____

   d. The child with appendicitis may exhibit guarding and rebound tenderness when the nurse performs an abdominal assessment. _____

35. How is nystatin (Mycostatin) applied to the mouth of a child with thrush? *(661, Nursing Tip, giving nystatin)* _____

   _____

36. What is the most common sign of pinworms? *(662)* _____

   _____

37. Describe the treatment of pinworms. *(662)* _____

   _____

   _____

   _____

   _____

38. The goals in the treatment of poisoning are: *(662)*

   a. _____

   b. _____

   c. _____

   d. _____

39. Activated charcoal should not be given with _____ because it will neutralize both, rendering both ineffective in the treatment of poisoning. *(663)*

40. An overdose of acetaminophen can result in _____ damage. *(663)*

41. The primary source of lead poisoning is _____. *(664; Box 28-1)*

42. Lead poisoning can have a lasting effect on the _____ system. *(666)*

43. Match each type of dehydration with its definition (a–c). *(657)*

_____ Hypotonic	a.	Loss of more electrolytes than water
_____ Hypertonic	b.	Loss of equal amounts of water and electrolytes
_____ Isotonic	c.	Loss of more water than electrolytes

44. Interpret the following arterial blood gas values to determine the acid-base imbalance. *(658; Table 28-5)*

a. _____   pH 7.32 $PaCO_2$ 37 HCO_3 20

b. _____   pH 7.48 $PaCO_2$ 33 HCO_3 24

REVIEW QUESTIONS

1. Which diagnostic test permits visualization of the upper GI tract? *(643)*
   1. Colonoscopy
   2. Sigmoidoscopy
   3. Endoscopy
   4. Proctoscopy

2. Children with failure to thrive fall below the _____ percentile in weight and height on growth charts. *(659)*
   1. 3rd
   2. 6th
   3. 10th
   4. 15th

3. Which approach might best support maternal attachment when caring for a child with failure to thrive? *(660)*
   1. Point out areas where the mother needs improvement.
   2. Send the mother to a parenting class.
   3. Encourage the mother to participate in the child's care.
   4. Leave the room when the mother visits.

4. Which signs and symptoms are characteristic of pinworms? *(662)*
   1. Diarrhea, itching, and fever
   2. Nausea, vomiting, and itching
   3. Nausea, vomiting, and weight loss
   4. Itching, irritability, and restlessness

5. Children with intussusception may have bowel movements containing blood and mucus and no feces. These are called: *(649)*
   1. currant jelly stools.
   2. mucoid stools.
   3. steatorrhea.
   4. occult blood stools.

6. A newborn's total body weight is about _____ water. *(655; Fig. 28-9)*
   1. 77%
   2. 60%
   3. 55%
   4. 45%

7. Which action should the nurse take before adding potassium to a child's IV? *(657; Safety Alert)*
   1. Take a baseline blood pressure.
   2. Determine if the child can tolerate oral fluids.
   3. Establish that the child is voiding.
   4. Place the child on a cardiac monitor.

8. The greatest threat to life in isotonic dehydration is: *(656; Table 28-2)*
   1. hypervolemic shock.
   2. hypovolemic shock.
   3. decreased K levels.
   4. clammy mucous membranes.

9. The nurse taking a history from parents of an infant with pyloric stenosis would expect them to report the infant experienced which sign? *(645)*
   1. Constipation
   2. Projectile vomiting
   3. Diarrhea
   4. Anorexia

10. When a child has pinworms, the nurse should know that: *(662)*
    1. a warm stool specimen must be sent to the lab.
    2. the child will be hospitalized for the duration of infection.
    3. any family member with symptoms should be treated.
    4. any pregnant household member must be treated with mebendazole.

11. Which information would the nurse give to parents of an infant with gastroesophageal reflux disease? *(651; Fig. 28-8)*
    1. Feed the infant half-strength formula.
    2. Position in an infant seat after feeding.
    3. Increase the time between feedings.
    4. Place in upright prone position after feeding.

12. The nurse doing a newborn assessment knows the earliest sign of Hirschsprung's disease is: *(648; Fig. 28-5)*
    1. failure to pass meconium.
    2. large, bulky, and frothy stools.
    3. acute, sudden diarrhea.
    4. ribbon-like stools.

13. The organ damaged by acetaminophen poisoning is the: *(665)*
    1. gallbladder.
    2. pancreas.
    3. liver.
    4. stomach.

14. The nurse should explain to parents that infants are more susceptible to accidental ingestion of foreign bodies because they are: *(667)*
    1. often left unattended.
    2. likely to put everything in their mouths.
    3. constantly hungry.
    4. seeking parental attention.

15. A nurse is giving a newborn her first feeding when the baby starts coughing and choking. This is indicative of which condition? *(644; Fig. 28-2)*
    1. Celiac disease
    2. Enterocolitis
    3. Tracheoesophageal atresia
    4. Pyloric stenosis

16. A child appears apathetic and weak. His growth is below normal for his age. There is a white streak in the child's hair. The nurse recognizes these signs as characteristic of: *(660; Fig. 28-10B)*
    1. rickets.
    2. scurvy.
    3. gastroesophageal reflux.
    4. kwashiorkor.

17. A child's arterial blood gas results are: pH 7.30, $PaCO_2$ 36, HCO_3 21. The nurse determines the child is experiencing which acid-base imbalance? *(658)*
    1. Respiratory acidosis
    2. Respiratory alkalosis
    3. Metabolic acidosis
    4. Metabolic alkalosis

CASE STUDY

1. Six-month-old Ava is diagnosed with failure to thrive. Ava's mother, Jenny, is a single mother who does not work outside the home. Neighbors report that they often hear Ava crying and that Jenny seldom holds her. They also report that Jenny has related to them that being a mother is not what she thought it would be.
    a. List some of the signs of failure to thrive that might be evident.
    b. What treatment for failure to thrive might be implemented?
    c. How would you involve Ava's mother in her care?
    d. Describe any of Jenny's behaviors that suggest postpartum depression. *(See Chapter 10, pp. 246-247)*
    e. Discuss your feelings toward parents who neglect their children. If Jenny is diagnosed with postpartum depression, does that alter your perception of her behaviors toward Ava? In what way?

THINKING CRITICALLY

1. You are speaking to a parent whose child has mild diarrhea. The parent explains that she has been giving the child a BRAT diet. Is this an appropriate intervention? If not, what will you recommend for this child?

2. You are caring for a child who drank a poisonous substance. What feelings might the child's parents be having? How can you assist the parents?

APPLYING KNOWLEDGE

1. Observe an endoscopy (if possible) on a child or adult.

2. Use Figure 28-1 in the textbook to describe the following.
    a. Functions of each portion of the GI tract
    b. Functions performed by the glands
    c. Aspects of chemical versus mechanical food breakdown
    d. Differences in these functions between child and adult

3. Develop a teaching plan related to poison prevention.

4. Develop a teaching plan related to parent care of a child with diarrhea.

The Child with a Genitourinary Condition

Answer Key: A complete answer key can be found on the Student Evolve website.

LEARNING ACTIVITIES

1. Match the terms in the left column with their definitions on the right (a–j).

   _____ Cystitis *(674)*

   _____ Frequency *(672)*

   _____ Hydrocele *(680)*

   _____ Hypospadias *(672; Fig. 29-6)*

   _____ Oliguria *(672)*

   _____ Phimosis *(672)*

   _____ Polyuria *(672)*

   _____ Pyelonephritis *(674)*

   _____ Urgency *(672)*

   _____ Vesicoureteral reflux *(674)*

   a. Backward flow of urine into the ureters
   b. Abnormal number of voidings in a short period of time
   c. Inflammation of the bladder
   d. Infection of the kidney and pelvis
   e. Excessive amount of fluid in the scrotal sac
   f. Decreased urinary output
   g. Narrowing of the preputial opening of the foreskin
   h. Impulse to void but inability to do so
   i. Congenital defect in which the urinary meatus is not at the end of the penis but on the lower shaft
   j. Increased urinary output

2. List five tests used to determine the cause of urinary dysfunction. *(672; Table 29-1)*

   a. _____

   b. _____

   c. _____

   d. _____

   e. _____

3. True or false?

   a. The newborn's kidneys function immaturely. *(669; Fig. 29-1)* _____

   b. There is an unexplained relationship between low-set ears and anomalies of the urinary tract. *(670)* _____

   c. Phimosis is normal in newborn males and usually disappears by the time a boy is 3 years old. *(672)* _____

   d. The optimal time for surgical repair of hypospadias and epispadias is in the late preschool period. *(673; Fig. 29-6)* _____

   e. Surgical repair of exstrophy of the bladder is done in the first 2 days of life. *(673)* _____

4. Distention of the renal pelvis due to an obstruction is referred to as _____. *(673)*

5. How would the nurse assess a child for bladder distention? *(674)* _____

    _____

    _____

6. List four of the possible reasons why urinary tract infections (UTIs) are more common in girls than in boys. *(674; Nursing Care Plan 29-1)*

    a. _____

    b. _____

    c. _____

    d. _____

7. What laboratory test is done to confirm a diagnosis of UTI? *(675)* _____

    _____

    _____

8. What classification of medication is used to treat a newly identified UTI in a 4-year-old child? *(675)*

    _____

9. a. The characteristic sign of nephrotic syndrome is _____. *(675)*

    b. Where does this usually occur first? *(675)* _____

10. The nurse would expect a urinalysis of a child with nephrotic syndrome to reveal massive _____. *(675)*

11. What is the treatment of choice for nephrotic syndrome? *(675, 677)* _____

    _____

12. List three types of positioning care that might be given to a child with nephrotic syndrome. *(677)*

    a. _____

    b. _____

    c. _____

13. When observing the urine of a child with nephrotic syndrome, the nurse should note: *(677, Nursing Tip)*

    a. _____

    b. _____

    c. _____

    d. _____

14. The child receiving treatment for nephrotic syndrome is at risk for _____. *(676)*

15. Acute glomerulonephritis is thought to be a(n) _____ reaction caused by _____. *(677; Table 29-3)*

16. List four nursing interventions that would be appropriate for the child who has acute glomerulonephritis. *(678)*

    a. _____

    b. _____

    c. _____

    d. _____

17. Foods high in _____ are restricted when a child with acute glomerulonephritis is oliguric. *(678)*

18. What organ is affected by Wilms' tumor? *(678)* _____

19. What is involved in the treatment of Wilms' tumor? *(679)*

    a. _____

    b. _____

    c. _____

20. What precaution is taken in a child with a Wilms' tumor to prevent spread of the disease? *(679, Safety Alert)*

    _____

21. Cryptorchidism with acute scrotal pain can indicate a condition called _____. *(681)*

22. Surgical repair of cryptorchidism is called _____. *(681)*

REVIEW QUESTIONS

1. The nurse planning care for a child with nephrotic syndrome knows the classification of medication used to reduce edema in nephrotic syndrome is: *(675)*
    1. fungicide.
    2. antibiotics.
    3. analgesics.
    4. steroids.

2. An expected outcome for a child with nephrotic syndrome is the prevention of: *(677)*
    1. skin breakdown.
    2. an antigen–antibody reaction.
    3. pathologic fractures.
    4. urinary stasis.

3. Which statement indicates to the nurse that a parent understands information about hypospadias? *(673)*
    1. "This defect must be corrected in the first 48 hours of life."
    2. "Fertility will most likely be reduced."
    3. "The condition usually resolves by the third birthday."
    4. "Surgical repair is usually performed by age 18 months."

4. Which instructions should the nurse give parents about caring for a child with acute glomerulonephritis with oliguria? *(678)*
   1. No restrictions on activity
   2. Remain on bedrest for 2 weeks
   3. Limit activity until gross hematuria subsides
   4. Encourage a diet high in potassium (e.g., bananas)

5. The nurse should assess a child with acute glomerulonephritis for the presence of: *(678)*
   1. urinary frequency.
   2. petechiae.
   3. hypotension.
   4. hypertension.

6. Wilms' tumors are often discovered when: *(678)*
   1. children enter school.
   2. the child has flank pain.
   3. blood is noted in the urine.
   4. a routine physical is given.

7. A parent reports her son's urethral opening is located on the undersurface of the penis. The nurse recognizes the child has which genitourinary condition? *(672; Fig. 29-6B)*
   1. Hydrocele
   2. Phimosis
   3. Hypospadias
   4. Cryptorchidism

8. What information should the nurse include when teaching young girls about preventing UTIs? *(675, Nursing Tip)*
   1. Wear nylon underwear.
   2. Void only when the bladder is full.
   3. Limit fluids after 8:00 PM.
   4. Wipe from front to back.

9. The etiology of acute glomerulonephritis is thought to be a(n): *(677; Table 29-3)*
   1. antigen–antibody reaction.
   2. autoimmune disease.
   3. malignant disease.
   4. infectious disease.

10. The nurse assessing urinary output for a child with acute glomerulonephritis should expect urine to be: *(678)*
    1. straw-colored.
    2. smoky brown.
    3. cloudy and concentrated.
    4. yellow with many mucous shreds.

11. Which is a sign of a UTI in a 6-year-old child? *(675, 676, Nursing Care Plan 29-1)*
    1. Proteinuria
    2. Perineal rash
    3. Hematuria
    4. Pain during urination

12. The nurse is caring for a child who has a ureterostomy. With this urinary diversion the nurse is aware: *(Table 29-2, 674)*
    1. the ureters were removed from the bladder and attached to the colon.
    2. an opening was created into the bladder between the umbilicus and pubis.
    3. ureters are surgically implanted outside the abdominal wall.
    4. a tube was passed through the flank into the pelvis of kidney.

13. Children receiving steroids for nephrosis should be: *(677; Safety Alert, 677)*
    1. placed on antibiotics before there are signs of an infection.
    2. isolated from other children receiving steroids.
    3. monitored closely for signs of infection.
    4. taken off the medication after 1 week.

14. When weighing diapers on a gram scale, the conversion from grams to milliliters is: *(677)*
    1. 1 g = 2.5 mL.
    2. 1 g = 1 mL.
    3. 1 g = 0.5 mL.
    4. 1 g = 0.25 mL.

15. While the child with nephrotic syndrome is being treated, he or she should not receive: *(677)*
    1. antihistamines.
    2. immunizations.
    3. diuretics.
    4. analgesics.

16. While caring for a child with glomerulonephritis, the nurse observes a rise in the child's blood pressure. What is the most appropriate nursing action? *(678)*
    1. Document the change.
    2. Recheck the blood pressure regularly.
    3. Notify the physician.
    4. Restrict sodium and fluid intake.

17. What is an acceptable urine output for an 18-month-old child? *(669; 682, Key Points)*
    1. 4-5 mL/kg/hr
    2. 2-3 mL/kg/hr
    3. 1-2 mL/kg/hr
    4. 0.5-1 mL/kg/hr

18. What nursing action would be avoided when caring for a child diagnosed with Wilms' tumor? *(679)*
    1. Measuring urinary output
    2. Monitoring blood pressure
    3. Abdominal palpation
    4. Auscultation of lungs

19. A parent tells the nurse, "My child is going to have a test that takes an x-ray before and while he is urinating." The child is scheduled for which diagnostic study? *(671)*
    1. Voiding cystourethrography
    2. Cystoscopy
    3. Cystometrogram
    4. Uroflow study

CROSSWORD PUZZLE

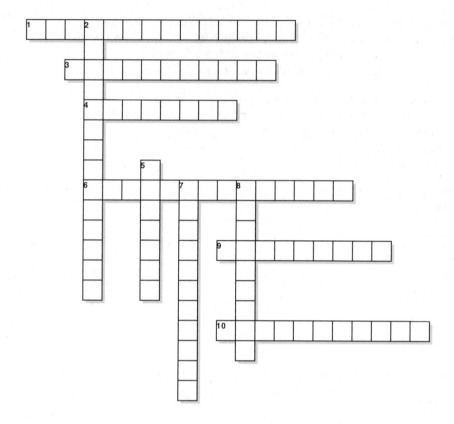

Across

1. Undescended testicle *(681)*
3. Surgical opening into the bladder between the umbilicus and pubis *(674, Table 29-2)*
4. Decreased urinary output *(672)*
6. Distention of the renal pelvis caused by obstruction *(673)*
9. Abnormal number of voidings in a short period *(672)*
10. Protein in the blood *(675)*

Down

2. Infection of the kidney and renal pelvis *(674)*
5. Urge to void but inability to do so *(672)*
7. Absolute neutrophil count below 1000/mm³ *(677)*
8. Excessive amount of fluid in the sac that surrounds the testicle *(680)*

CASE STUDY

1. Three-year-old Tucker is hospitalized with nephrotic syndrome. He is pale, lethargic, anorexic, and has generalized edema.
   a. Tucker is put on steroid therapy. What are three nursing interventions associated with his treatment?
   b. Plan a menu for Tucker for one day using the nutritional requirements necessary for his recovery.
   c. Tucker likes to lie on his stomach. When you change his position, he is irritable and his mother objects. What would you tell his mother?

THINKING CRITICALLY

1. A child you are caring for is in renal failure as a result of chronic glomerulonephritis. She is being evaluated for a kidney transplant. Use the library to research this topic. Include in your information the selection process, procedure, risks, expense, recovery, and maintenance.

2. Identify foods that are low in potassium for a child or adult who should limit this electrolyte. Search a nutrition text or the Internet. State the source of your information about foods that may be included in a low-potassium diet.

APPLYING KNOWLEDGE

1. Use Figure 29-1 in the textbook to label the following.

   a. Kidney
   b. Ureter
   c. Urinary bladder
   d. Urethra

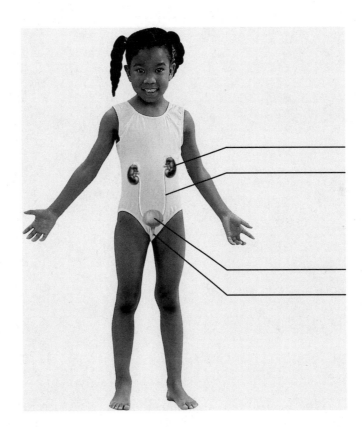

2. While in the clinical area, collect a urine specimen for urinalysis from an infant and a toddler.

3. Measure abdominal girth on a child with ascites. What indicates correct level for this measurement?

4. Keep an intake and output record on a child with a genitourinary condition.

Student Name_____   Date_____

The Child with a Skin Condition

chapter
30

Answer Key: A complete answer key can be found on the Student Evolve website.

LEARNING ACTIVITIES

1. Match the terms in the left column with their definitions on the right (a–j).

    _____ Comedo *(688; Fig. 30-9)*
    _____ Débridement *(698)*
    _____ Exanthem *(684)*
    _____ Heterograft *(698)*
    _____ Homograft *(698)*
    _____ Isograft *(698)*
    _____ Miliaria *(686)*
    _____ Pruritus *(686)*
    _____ Strawberry nevus *(684, Figure 30-3)*
    _____ Wheal *(685, Box 30-1)*

    a. Benign hemangioma that disappears without treatment
    b. Graft tissue from a source other than human
    c. Removal of dried crusts
    d. Graft tissue from cadavers
    e. Irregular red, raised area associated with allergic reactions
    f. Plug of keratin, sebum, or bacteria
    g. Skin rash
    h. Graft from the patient's identical twin
    i. Itching
    j. Rash caused by excess body heat and moisture

2. Identify at least three tests useful in diagnosing a skin condition. *(684)* _____

    _____

    _____

    _____

3. List at least three of the possible characteristics to describe skin lesions. *(684)*

    a. _____

    b. _____

    c. _____

4. What is miliaria? What is another common name for the condition? *(686, Figure 30-5)* _____

    _____

5. How can intertrigo be prevented? *(687)* _____

    _____

6. How would the nurse advise parents about the treatment for an infant who has seborrheic dermatitis? What is another common name for this condition? *(687; Fig. 30-7)*

_____

_____

_____

_____

_____

7. How can diaper dermatitis be prevented? What is a common name for the condition? *(687, Figure 30-8)*

_____

_____

_____

_____

_____

8. Briefly describe the pathology of acne. *(688)* _____

_____

_____

9. Eczema is actually a(n) _____, rather than a disorder. *(689)*

10. The main contraindication for anyone taking Accutane is _____ _____. *(688)*

11. A medication that may reduce viral shedding and hasten healing of herpes simplex type 1 infection is topical _____. *(689)*

12. Eczema is indicative of _____. *(689)*

13. Allergens enter the body of the child with eczema through: *(689)*

a. _____

b. _____

c. _____

d. _____

14. Describe the application of ointment to the skin of a child with eczema. *(689-690)*_____

_____

_____

_____

15. The organism responsible for causing scalded skin syndrome is _____. *(692)*

16. What is impetigo? *(692; Fig. 30-12)* _____

_____

17. How can impetigo be prevented? *(692-693)* _____

_____

_____

18. Describe the treatment of impetigo. *(693)* _____

_____

_____

_____

19. Identify the body parts affected in the following tinea infections and other names they may be called. *(693)*

   a.   Tinea capitis: _____

   b.   Tinea corporis: _____

   c.   Tinea pedis: _____

   d.   Tinea cruris: _____

20. Describe the drug treatment of tinea capitis and parent-child teaching that should be done. *(693)*

_____

_____

_____

21. True or false? *(693)*

   a.   Tinea occurs when fungus invades the hair, the stratum corneum layer of the skin, or the nails. _____

   b.   Tinea infections are not contagious to others. _____

   c.   Tinea pedis heals more quickly if the affected area is kept warm and moist. _____

22. The main symptom of pediculosis is _____. *(694)*

23. The most common form of pediculosis infestation is _____. *(694)*

24. What are scabies? *(694)* _____

_____

_____

25. List the four types of burns and their causes. *(695)*

    a. _____

    b. _____

    c. _____

    d. _____

26. When a child is burned by fire near the face, assessing for _____ and _____ _____ is a priority. *(695, Safety Alert)*

27. The severity of a burn depends on the _____, _____, and _____ of involvement. *(695)*

28. Match the burn classification with the correct description (a–c). *(696; Table 30-2)*

    _____ Superficial

    _____ Partial thickness

    _____ Full thickness

    a. Blistered, moist, pink, or red; painful
    b. Tough, leathery, dry; painless to touch
    c. Skin red but blanches easily and refills quickly; painful

29. Indications that flames may have been inhaled include: *(695)*

    a. _____

    b. _____

    c. _____

    d. _____

30. If eschar from burns on the trunk inhibits respirations, a(n) _____ is made in order to prevent restriction of chest movement. *(697)*

31. Urine output is observed _____ in a burn patient. *(698)*

32. What is the rationale for inserting a nasogastric tube into a burn patient? *(698)* _____

    _____

    _____

33. Describe how a burn wound is dressed. *(699; Fig. 30-17)* _____

    _____

    _____

    _____

    _____

34. Describe how protective isolation is instituted with a burn patient. *(700)* _____

_____

_____

_____

_____

35. List the signs and symptoms of infection in a burn patient. *(700)*

a. _____

b. _____

c. _____

d. _____

e. _____

36. What type of diet should a burn patient be given? *(700)* _____

_____

_____

_____

37. Analgesics are administered _____ painful procedures, such as dressing changes. *(700)*

38. a. What type of light rays are absorbed by a sunscreen? _____

    b. What does the acronym *SPF* refer to? _____ *(701)*

39. The school nurse is talking with children about preventing frostbite. What should be included in the nurse's explanation about dressing for outdoor activities? *(701)*

_____

_____

REVIEW QUESTIONS

1. Which of the following skin conditions is *not* contagious? *(689)*
   1. Impetigo
   2. *Staphylococcus aureus* infection
   3. Infantile eczema
   4. Pediculosis

2. What information would the nurse give to parents about the treatment of pediculosis capitis? *(694)*
   1. All family members must be treated.
   2. Wash the child's hair with hydrogen peroxide.
   3. Apply prescription lotion to the entire body.
   4. Use a fine-toothed comb to remove nits.

3. The nurse determines a parent understands instructions when she tells the nurse first-aid treatment of a partial-thickness burn should include: *(696)*
   1. application of butter.
   2. immersion in cold water.
   3. maintaining exposure to clean air.
   4. breaking the blisters.

4. A full-thickness burn can best be described as: *(696; Table 30-2)*
   1. red with good refill, painful.
   2. mottled, red, dull white, painful.
   3. blistered, pink or red, painful.
   4. tough, leathery, painless to touch.

5. The nurse assessing a child with burns recognizes which finding as an early sign of sepsis? *(700; Nursing Tip)*
   1. Decreased pulse
   2. Erythema
   3. Elevated temperature
   4. Decreased blood pressure

6. A burn patient with cyanosis and charred lips may need a(n): *(697)*
   1. nasogastric tube.
   2. endotracheal tube.
   3. Foley catheter.
   4. throat culture.

7. The priority goal in the management of a severe burn is: *(697)*
   1. wound débridement.
   2. pain control.
   3. fluid replacement.
   4. airway maintenance.

8. The nurse would teach parents of a child with impetigo to be alert for signs of which complication? *(693)*
   1. Rheumatoid arthritis
   2. Nephritis
   3. Endocarditis
   4. Otitis media

9. The nurse would instruct an adolescent who is taking Accutane to avoid: *(688)*
   1. sun exposure.
   2. dairy products.
   3. pregnancy.
   4. strenuous exercise.

10. When inspecting children for pediculosis capitis, special attention should be paid to which area of the body? *(694)*
    1. Pubic area
    2. Hairline at the back of the neck
    3. Bottoms of the feet
    4. Underarms

11. A common manifestation of an allergy in a neonate is: *(689)*
    1. port wine stain.
    2. infantile eczema.
    3. strawberry nevus.
    4. Mongolian spots.

12. What is the most appropriate nursing response to an adolescent who asks what she can do about her acne? *(688)*
    1. "Restrict the amount of chocolate and peanuts you eat."
    2. "Wash your face at least four times a day."
    3. "Get adequate rest and eat a well-balanced diet."
    4. "Stay out of the sun even if you are not on medication."

13. The nurse is caring for a child who received a skin graft from pigskin. This type of graft is called a(n): *(698)*
    1. homograft.
    2. heterograft.
    3. isograft.
    4. autograft.

14. A priority in changing the dressing of a burn patient is: *(700)*
    1. asking the parents to leave the room.
    2. medicating for pain prior to the procedure.
    3. limiting the number of dressing changes.
    4. doing the procedure in the child's room.

15. A child who has been burned eats only a small amount of the food on her tray. An appropriate nursing action would be to: *(700)*
    1. request an order to start an IV.
    2. insert a nasogastric tube for feeding.
    3. offer the child small, frequent feedings.
    4. leave the tray at the bedside longer.

16. Scabies are most strongly characterized by: *(694)*
    1. round, dry patches on the arms.
    2. intense itching.
    3. a purulent drainage.
    4. round lesions similar to chickenpox.

17. A topical ointment is prescribed for an infant with eczema. Which application strategy is key to maximizing its absorption? *(689-690)*
    1. Apply a generous amount of ointment to affected areas.
    2. Use a circular motion to massage the ointment into the skin.
    3. Keep the fingernails short to prevent scratching the infant.
    4. For best absorption, apply ointment after bathing the child.

18. You work at a pediatric clinic and develop a cold sore, or herpes zoster, while at work. Which of these children should you avoid contacting directly to prevent complications to the child? *(689)*
    1. 10-month-old girl with allergies and diagnosed as infantile eczema
    2. 18-month-old boy showing generalized rash after starting antibiotics
    3. 2-month-old boy showing dermatitis in area of wet diaper
    4. 5-year-old girl diagnosed with pediculosis by school nurse

CASE STUDIES

1. Stacey, a 17-year-old teenager diagnosed with acne vulgaris, is prescribed Accutane because other medications have not been effective.
    a. What can the nurse tell Stacey about the side effects of isotretinoin (Accutane)?
    b. What is the pregnancy category for isotretinoin? Check your drug reference.

    c.   Check Food and Drug Administration (FDA) for expected monitoring of isotretinoin. Also available at http://aapnews.aappublications.org/cgi/content/full/26/2/23 for online information. Print publication: AAP News. (2005). FDA strengthens monitoring of acne drug isotretinoin, 26(2), p. 23.

    d.   Stacey asks if there is anything she can do with her diet to improve the acne. What should the nurse tell her?

    e.   What are some topical preparations that could be recommended for Stacey's acne?

2.   Ten-month-old Taylor is admitted to the hospital with a diagnosis of atopic dermatitis. His face, arms, and legs are erythematous and are covered with vesicles, some of which have crusted over. The physician's orders include a soy-based formula, addition of therapeutic bath oil to soften Taylor's dry and crusted skin, cut his fingernails, and place in private room.

    a.   What is infantile eczema (atopic dermatitis)?

    b.   What does the order for a soy-based formula have to do with Taylor's diagnosis?

    c.   Explain rationale for each of the orders listed.

    d.   Describe parent teaching about care of atopic dermatitis.

    e.   Taylor is irritable and continually attempts to scratch his arms and legs. What can the nurse do to soothe him?

THINKING CRITICALLY

1.   Use the nursing process to plan care for a 9-year-old child who was admitted to the hospital with full-thickness burns of the chest and arms 2 days ago. He is burned over 15% of his body. His treatment plan includes an IV, reverse isolation, occlusive dressings with Silvadene to the wound, regular diet with high-protein feedings between meals, and morphine for pain. What do you consider to be the four most important nursing diagnoses? State expected outcomes of care and nursing interventions for one nursing diagnosis. Compare your care plan with others'.

APPLYING KNOWLEDGE

1.   When you are in the clinical setting, read the charts and find a description of skin on:

    a.   an admission assessment.

    b.   a child with a skin disorder.

    c.   a child with a burn.

The Child with a Metabolic Condition

Answer Key: A complete answer key can be found on the Student Evolve website.

LEARNING ACTIVITIES

1. Match the terms in the left column with their definitions on the right (a–g).

    _____ Glycosuria *(708)*

    _____ Hormones *(703)*

    _____ Hyperglycemia *(708)*

    _____ Hypoglycemia *(715; Table 31-4)*

    _____ Kussmaul's respirations *(709; Table 31-4)*

    _____ Polydipsia *(708)*

    _____ Polyphagia *(708)*

    a. Excessive thirst
    b. Constant hunger
    c. Higher-than-normal glucose in the blood
    d. Lower-than-normal glucose in the blood
    e. Glucose in the urine
    f   Type of respirations seen in diabetic ketoacidosis
    g. Chemical substances produced by glands

2. Identify five early signs of inborn errors of metabolism in a newborn. *(703)*

    a. _____

    b. _____

    c. _____

    d. _____

    e. _____

3. The pattern of inheritance for inborn errors of metabolism is most often _____ _____. *(704)*

4. _____ testing and _____ counseling have markedly decreased the occurrence of Tay-Sachs disease. *(705)*

5. List five or more manifestations of hypothyroidism. *(705)*

    a. _____

    b. _____

    c. _____

    d. _____

    e. _____

6. What is essential to prevent permanent sequelae associated with congenital hypothyroidism? *(705)*

   _____

7. What information would the nurse give to parents about medication for the treatment of hypothyroidism? *(705)*

   _____

   _____

8. Describe the pathophysiology of diabetes insipidus. *(705)* _____

   _____

9. The initial signs of diabetes insipidus are _____ and _____. *(705)*

10. What would the nurse teach parents about administering DDAVP nasal spray to a child with diabetes insipidus? *(706)*

    _____

    _____

    _____

11. Describe the pathophysiology of diabetes mellitus. *(706)* _____

    _____

    _____

    _____

12. Type 1 diabetes mellitus is considered to be a(n) _____ disease. *(707)*

13. Type 2 diabetes mellitus involves a(n) _____ to insulin. *(707)*

14. The onset of type 1 diabetes mellitus is increased in pubescent children. Give two possible causes of this increase. *(707)*

    a. _____

    b. _____

15. What are the three "Ps" of type 1 diabetes mellitus? *(708)*

    a. _____

    b. _____

    c. _____

16. What is the most reliable test to diagnose diabetes mellitus? *(708)* _____

    _____

17. What test measures glycemic levels over a period of months? *(709)* _____

    _____

18. List the three goals of treatment in type 1 diabetes mellitus. *(709)*

    a. _____

    b. _____

    c. _____

19. Children with diabetes mellitus have problems associated with their stage of growth and development. Give at least one example of a problem for each age group. *(709-710)*

    a. Infant: _____

    _____

    b. Toddler: _____

    _____

    c. Preschool child: _____

    _____

    d. School-age child: _____

    _____

    e. Adolescent: _____

    _____

20. List three goals of nutritional management for the child with type 1 diabetes mellitus. *(709)*

    a. _____

    _____

    b. _____

    _____

    c. _____

    _____

21. The standard form of insulin is _____. *(713)*

22. Describe insulin injection site rotation. *(713; Figure 31-5)* _____

    _____

    _____

    _____

    _____

    _____

23. List three reasons why a child is more prone to insulin shock than an adult. *(716)*

    a. _____

    b. _____

    c. _____

24. What is the immediate treatment for a child suspected of having an insulin reaction? *(716)*

    _____

    _____

25. _____ is recommended for the treatment of severe hypoglycemia. *(716)*

26. Explain the Somogyi phenomenon. *(716)* _____

    _____

    _____

    _____

27. List two precautions in the foot care of a child with diabetes. *(716)*

    a. _____

    b. _____

28. When a child with diabetes plans to travel, what should be done prior to and during the trip? *(717-718)*

    a. _____

    b. _____

    c. _____

    d. _____

29. Match each sign or symptom with its cause. *(Causes will be used more than once.) (709; Table 31-4)*

    _____ Fruity breath   a. Hypoglycemia
    _____ Headache   b. Hyperglycemia
    _____ Diaphoresis
    _____ Abdominal pain
    _____ Tremors
    _____ Deep, rapid respirations

30. True or false?

    a. The symptoms of diabetes mellitus appear more slowly in children. *(707-708; 716)* _____

    b. Exercise lowers blood glucose levels. *(709; Table 31-4)* _____

    c. Water intake should be limited for the child with diabetes insipidus. *(709, 711)* _____

    d. Children with type 1 diabetes mellitus require special foods. *(707)* _____

e. The child with type 1 diabetes mellitus is able to participate in almost all sports activities. *(711)* _____

f. If left untreated, congenital hypothyroidism can result in intellectual disability. *(705)* _____

g. When mixing insulin, the nurse draws up the longer-acting insulin into the syringe first. *(715, Medication Safety Alert)* _____

h. Human insulin manufactured by biosynthesis is the treatment of choice for type 1 diabetes mellitus. *(714)* _____

REVIEW QUESTIONS

1. The "honeymoon period" after diagnosis of type 1 diabetes in the child may result in: *(708; Nursing Tip)*
   1. parental denial of child's need for lifetime insulin.
   2. return of child's weight gain to the previous level.
   3. brief period with no food restrictions needed.
   4. more active exercise with increased insulin available.

2. In general, a child can be taught to perform self-injection after the age of: *(714, Fig. 31-7B)*
   1. 7 years.
   2. 3 years.
   3. 5 years.
   4. 13 years.

3. An initial sign of diabetes insipidus is: *(705)*
   1. polyphagia.
   2. polydipsia.
   3. excessive perspiration.
   4. hyperglycemia.

4. What is the best immediate food choice for the nurse to give to a child having an insulin reaction? *(716)*
   1. Orange juice
   2. Unsalted crackers
   3. Diet soda
   4. Apple slices

5. The nurse recognizes a sign of diabetic ketoacidosis is: *(709, Table 31-4)*
   1. hyperactivity.
   2. increased heart rate.
   3. deep, rapid respirations.
   4. blue lips and fingertips.

6. The most common concentration of insulin is: *(713)*
   1. U35 insulin.
   2. U40 insulin.
   3. U80 insulin.
   4. U100 insulin.

7. The nurse determines a parent understands teaching about hypoglycemia when he identifies which as a cause of hypoglycemia in children? *(716)*
   1. Eating too much food
   2. Using insufficient insulin
   3. Gastrointestinal illness
   4. Poorly planned exercise

8. The nurse recognizes a child with type 1 diabetes mellitus is having an insulin reaction when which sign occurs? *(716)*
    1. Dry skin and anorexia
    2. Flushed face and red hands
    3. Irritable, pale, and weak
    4. Increased thirst and passivity

9. Regular insulin is considered: *(714, Table 31-6)*
    1. short-acting.
    2. rapid-acting.
    3. intermediate-acting.
    4. long-acting.

10. A characteristic common to type 1 diabetes mellitus is that it: *(707)*
    1. is more common in preschool-age children.
    2. is often seen in obese individuals.
    3. always requires insulin therapy.
    4. has few blood sugar fluctuations.

11. What information would the nurse include when speaking to expectant parents about Tay-Sachs disease? *(705)*
    1. Only the mother passes the disease to the child.
    2. There is no known cause for this disease.
    3. There is a positive outcome if diagnosed before age 6 months.
    4. Carriers can be identified by a screening test.

12. The nurse would teach a child with type 1 diabetes mellitus to check urine for acetone when he: *(717)*
    1. is exercising.
    2. is sick.
    3. eats meals.
    4. has a growth spurt.

13. Screening for hypothyroidism is done for all infants: *(705)*
    1. of high-risk families.
    2. at 6 months of age.
    3. at birth.
    4. at 2 weeks of age.

14. What information would the nurse include in teaching about thyroid hormone replacement for children with hypothyroidism? *(705)*
    1. It may cause excessive hair growth on the body.
    2. Medication is continued for the duration of the child's life.
    3. The full effect may not be reached for 3 months.
    4. Signs of overdosage include lethargy and constipation.

15. The nurse determines a parent of a child with diabetes insipidus requires additional teaching when she says a sign of water intoxication is: *(706)*
    1. polyuria.
    2. edema.
    3. nausea.
    4. lethargy.

16. The nurse teaching parents about type 2 diabetes mellitus would explain that it is associated with insulin: *(707)*
    1. overproduction.
    2. sensitivity.
    3. deficiency.
    4. resistance.

CASE STUDY

1. Alexa, 16 years old, is newly diagnosed with type 1 diabetes mellitus. She is a cheerleader and plays basketball. Since her diagnosis, Alexa's parents are constantly with Alexa and are very protective of her.
   a. Alexa asks if she has to eat special foods. What should the nurse tell Alexa about nutritional management of diabetes mellitus?
   b. Alexa asks if she can still play basketball and remain a cheerleader. What should the nurse tell her about these activities?
   c. Alexa becomes very impatient with her mother and accuses her of hovering. How can emotional turmoil have an effect on an adolescent with diabetes mellitus?
   d. How should the nurse respond to Alexa when she asks, "How did I get diabetes?"

THINKING CRITICALLY

1. Plot a curve showing the peaks and duration of action for a child who is receiving a combination of regular and NPH insulin at 7:30 AM and 5:30 PM.

APPLYING KNOWLEDGE

1. While in the clinical area, teach a child or a parent to give insulin.

2. While in the clinical area, teach a family home glucose monitoring. Include the child if old enough.

3. Care for a child or adult in diabetic ketoacidosis.

Childhood Communicable Diseases, Bioterrorism, Natural Disasters, and the Maternal-Child Patient

Answer Key: A complete answer key can be found on the Student Evolve website.

LEARNING ACTIVITIES

1. Match the terms in the left column with their definitions on the right (a–h).

_____ Epidemic *(725)*	a. Interval between the earliest symptoms and the appearance of the rash or fever
_____ Erythema *(727)*	b. Inanimate material that absorbs and transmits infection
_____ Fomite *(725)*	c. Insect or animal that carries and spreads a disease
_____ Incubation period *(725)*	d. Sudden increase of a communicable disease in a localized area
_____ Pandemic *(725)*	e. Diffuse, reddened area on the skin
_____ Prodromal period *(725)*	f. Circular, reddened area on the skin that is elevated and contains fluid
_____ Vector *(725)*	g. Worldwide high incidence of a communicable disease
_____ Vesicle *(727)*	h. Time between invasion by a pathogen and the onset of symptoms

2. Define *communicable disease. (725)* _____

_____

3. The incubation period for varicella is _____. *(722, Health Promotion)*

4. How long is the child with varicella contagious? *(722, Health Promotion)* _____

5. Describe the appearance of the child with fifth disease. *(722, Health Promotion)* _____

_____

6. List the manifestations of infectious mononucleosis. *(722)*

a. _____

b. _____

c. _____

d. _____

7. Identify at least three actions that can be taken to prevent Lyme disease. *(724)*

   a. _____

   b. _____

   c. _____

8. Careful _____ _____ is basic and essential to contain infection. *(725)*

9. What is an opportunistic infection? *(725)* _____

   _____

   _____

10. A child developed a wound infection while he was hospitalized postoperatively. This is called a(n) _____ _____-_____ infection. *(726)*

11. List three factors related to host resistance to disease. *(725)*

    a. _____

    b. _____

    c. _____

12. Vaccines provide _____ immunity to disease. *(726)*

13. A child received tetanus serum to prevent lockjaw. This is an example of _____ immunity. *(726)*

14. The Centers for Disease Control recommends _____ precautions for all patients. This involves _____ _____ and the use of _____ _____. *(726)*

15. Identify at least three types of patients for whom contact precautions are necessary. *(726-727)*

    a. _____

    b. _____

    c. _____

16. A nurse enters the room of a child hospitalized with influenza; the patient is coughing frequently. As the nurse approaches, at what distance from this patient does the nurse require mask and gown? Why? *(727)*

    _____

    _____

    _____

17. a. When would a child need protective environment isolation precautions? *(727)* _____

       _____

    b. What do these precautions consist of? *(727)* _____

       _____

18. Match the following terms with the correct description (a–e). *(727)*

    _____ Macule
    _____ Papule
    _____ Vesicle
    _____ Pustule
    _____ Scab

    a. Dried pustule covered with a crust
    b. Circular, reddened area on the skin that is elevated and contains fluid
    c. Circular, reddened area on the skin
    d. Circular, reddened area on the skin that is elevated and contains pus
    e. Circular, reddened area on the skin that is elevated

19. a. Why are immunizations not administered to infants under 2 months of age? *(728, Nursing Tip)*

    _____

    _____

    b. What is sometimes an exception to this rule, and why? *(728)* _____

    _____

20. The _____ of vaccine administration influences the infant's ability to exhibit an optimum response. *(728)*

21. _____ should be available on units where immunizations are given in case of _____. *(729)*

22. List six contraindications to administration of a live virus vaccine. *(731)*

    a. _____

    b. _____

    c. _____

    d. _____

    e. _____

    f. _____

23. The occurrence of a sexually transmitted infection (STI) in a 9-year-old child suggests the possibility of _____ _____. *(739)*

24. List the three ways in which children can acquire the human immunodeficiency virus (HIV). *(741)*

    a. _____

    b. _____

    c. _____

25. Identify three nursing diagnoses for a toddler with AIDS. *(742; Nursing Care Plan 32-1)*

    a. _____

    b. _____

    c. _____

REVIEW QUESTIONS

1. Which disease does not require a routine immunization? *(721)*
   1. Chickenpox
   2. Smallpox
   3. Measles
   4. German measles

2. The period that refers to the initial stage of a disease between the earliest symptoms and the appearance of the rash or fever is the: *(725)*
   1. incubation period.
   2. infectious period.
   3. prodromal period.
   4. stage one period.

3. A child manifests signs and symptoms of respiratory syncytial virus (RSV) infection during a hospitalization for sickle cell crisis. This is referred to as a(n): *(726)*
   1. opportunistic infection.
   2. health care–associated infection.
   3. directly transmitted infection.
   4. pathognomonic infection.

4. A hospitalized child has varicella. The nurse arranges for which type of infection precautions? *(722)*
   1. Large droplet infection precautions
   2. Airborne infection precautions
   3. Contact precautions
   4. Indirect transmission precautions

5. While inspecting a child's skin, the nurse observes a circular, reddened area that is elevated and contains fluid. The nurse would document this finding as a: *(727)*
   1. vesicle.
   2. pustule.
   3. macule.
   4. papule.

6. A parent asks the nurse when her younger child will get chickenpox now that her oldest child contracted the illness. The nurse would explain the incubation period for chickenpox is: *(722)*
   1. 1–2 weeks after direct contact with varicella lesions.
   2. 4–14 days after direct exposure to brother's rash.
   3. 2–3 weeks after home exposure to brother with varicella.
   4. 15–45 days after brother's rash fades.

7. A child with pertussis would be placed in which type of isolation? *(723, 727)*
   1. Droplet precautions
   2. Airborne precautions
   3. Contact precautions
   4. Protective environment isolation precautions

8. The most important nursing action in preventing the spread of infection is: *(725)*
   1. the administration of antibiotics.
   2. placing all children in private rooms.
   3. good hand hygiene.
   4. good nutrition.

9. The nurse observes Koplik's spots in the mouth of a child. This finding is associated with which communicable disease? *(727)*
    1. Chickenpox
    2. Rubella
    3. Rubeola
    4. Mumps

10. The risk of secondary infection in communicable diseases is reduced by: *(722)*
    1. giving all children antibiotics.
    2. keeping fingernails short.
    3. forcing fluids.
    4. isolating the child.

11. The disease that causes a "slapped cheek" appearance is: *(722)*
    1. Lyme disease.
    2. roseola.
    3. measles.
    4. fifth disease.

12. To protect against mumps, a child should receive the initial measles, mumps, rubella (MMR) vaccine at: *(723)*
    1. 4 months.
    2. 6 months.
    3. 15 months.
    4. 24 months.

13. If a vaccination series is interrupted: *(731, Nursing Tip)*
    1. the series must start over.
    2. it continues without restarting the entire series.
    3. future vaccines are given 28 days apart until the child is caught up.
    4. the child must wait 6 months before restarting the series.

14. Which child should *not* receive a live virus vaccine? *(731)*
    1. Taking prednisone
    2. Has an STI
    3. Was born prematurely
    4. Has a seizure disorder

THINKING CRITICALLY

1. Four-month-old Orlando has come to the pediatrician's office for his well-child checkup. His mother tells you that Orlando's immunizations are up to date. Refer to the immunization schedule (see Figure 32-6) to determine which immunizations he should receive at this visit.

2. You are asked to care for an adolescent with pelvic inflammatory disease. You know that she has been sexually active and has a history of STIs (also called *sexually transmitted diseases* or *STDs*). Think about this situation and then write down your thoughts about this teenage girl.

APPLYING KNOWLEDGE

1. Contact your local health department for information about educating the public about STIs. Request pamphlets and other written materials.

2. Assist nurses in a public health clinic to administer immunizations.

The Child with an Emotional or Behavioral Condition

Answer Key: A complete answer key can be found on the Student Evolve website.

LEARNING ACTIVITIES

1. Match the terms in the left column with their definitions on the right (a–f).

   _____ Gateway substances *(754)*
   _____ Milieu therapy *(747)*
   _____ Psychosomatic *(748)*
   _____ Suicidal attempt *(753)*
   _____ Suicidal gestures *(753)*
   _____ Suicidal ideation *(753)*

   a. Thoughts about suicide
   b. Attempt at a suicidal-type action that does not result in injury
   c. Action that is seriously intended to cause death
   d. Physical and social environment provided for the child
   e. Alcohol and common household products that can be abused to achieve an altered state of consciousness
   f. Bodily dysfunctions that seem to have an emotional or mental basis

2. Identify three interventions that may be used in the treatment of emotional or behavioral conditions. *(747)*

   a. _____

   b. _____

   c. _____

3. Creating a(n) _____ _____ environment is basic to all forms of therapy. *(747)*

4. Identify three deviations parents might watch for in early (12–24 months) development that may be red flags for a type of autistic disorder. *(748)*

   a. _____

   b. _____

   c. _____

5. a. What therapies may be used to treat the autistic child? *(748)*_____

   _____

   _____

b. What is the goal of therapy for a child who is autistic? *(748)* _____

_____

c. What is the nurse's role in treating a child who is autistic? *(748)*_____

_____

6. a. In obsessive-compulsive disorder (OCD), what is the difference between an obsession and a compulsion? *(748)*

_____

_____

b. How does OCD differ in children versus adults? *(748)* _____

_____

7. a. Describe the nurse's role in assessing a child with obsessive-compulsive disorder. *(749)*_____

_____

_____

b. How might a nurse reassure parents about the potential normalcy of ritualistic behavior in a 3-year-old? *(749)*

_____

_____

8. Describe five common signs and symptoms experienced by adolescents who are depressed. *(752)*

a. _____

b. _____

c. _____

d. _____

e. _____

9. The presence of which three factors increases the likelihood that a suicide attempt by an adolescent will be successful? *(753, Nursing Tip, Safety Alert)*

a. _____

b. _____

c. _____

10. Manifestations of suicidal behavior include: *(754; Safety Alert)*

    a. _____

    b. _____

    c. _____

    d. _____

    e. _____

    f. _____

11. True or false? *(752, Safety Alert; Nursing Tip, 754)*

    a. The nurse must take every threat of suicide seriously. _____

    b. When an adolescent feels hopeless and talks about feeling useless or worthless, it is important to immediately prove him or her wrong. _____

12. What are the four levels of substance abuse? *(754)*

    a. _____

    b. _____

    c. _____

    d. _____

13. What are the two types of drug dependence? *(754)*

    a. _____

    b. _____

14. List two strategies for the prevention of substance abuse. *(756-757)*

    a. _____

       _____

    b. _____

       _____

15. What is a gateway substance? *(754-755)* _____

    _____

16. The most significant consequence of heroin abuse is the increased risk of _____
    _____. *(756)*

17. Give two examples of each of the following clinical manifestations of a child with attention deficit hyperactivity disorder (ADHD). *(756; Nursing Tip)*

    a. Inattention: _____

    _____

    b. Impulsivity: _____

    _____

    c. Hyperactivity: _____

    _____

18. Describe the management of ADHD. *(749)*_____

    _____

    _____

19. The nurse can help a family cope with ADHD by emphasizing the child's _____ rather than the _____. *(Health Promotion, 749)*

20. The primary symptom of anorexia nervosa is severe _____ _____. *(750)*

21. List five of the possible body changes associated with anorexia nervosa. *(750)*

    a. _____

    b. _____

    c. _____

    d. _____

    e. _____

22. Describe at least three of the common behaviors of families of children with anorexia nervosa. *(750)*

    _____

    _____

    _____

    _____

23. Describe the eating habits of an adolescent with bulimia. *(751)* _____

    _____

    _____

24. Siblings of children with a long-term emotional disorders are at risk for developing poor _____-_____ and problems with _____ _____. *(758)*

REVIEW QUESTIONS

1. The risk of death increases in a suicidal adolescent when: *(753)*
    1. he is under pressure to succeed at school.
    2. he has a learning disorder.
    3. he has a plan of action.
    4. his parents are divorced.

2. The nurse talking with school-age children about alcohol should explain this substance is known to be a: *(755, Table 33-1)*
    1. sedative.
    2. opiate.
    3. stimulant.
    4. amphetamine.

3. Marijuana has which of the following physical effects? *(751, Table 33-1)*
    1. Respiratory depression
    2. Pupil dilation
    3. Anorexia
    4. Tachycardia

4. The street name for a form of cocaine is: *(754, Table 33-2)*
    1. speed.
    2. smack.
    3. hash.
    4. crack.

5. Primary to prevention of substance abuse in children is a: *(756)*
    1. positive self-image.
    2. strong religious belief.
    3. strict family.
    4. good education.

6. Adolescents who seek help for a substance abuse problem usually do so because: *(757)*
    1. there are no other options.
    2. they have friends in treatment.
    3. they realize they need help.
    4. their family encourages them.

7. If a nurse suspects an adolescent is contemplating suicide, he or she should: *(752, Nursing Care Plan 33-1)*
    1. avoid discussing the topic.
    2. ask the parents if they agree.
    3. ask the adolescent directly if he or she is thinking of killing him- or herself.
    4. observe him or her closely.

8. The best nursing response to a depressed adolescent is: *(753; Nursing Tip, 754)*
    1. "Cheer up, things will get better."
    2. "Let's talk about how you are feeling."
    3. "Things always seem worse than they are."
    4. "You are lucky to have so many friends."

9. The type of drug dependence that causes withdrawal symptoms is called: *(754)*
    1. psychological.
    2. emotional.
    3. physical.
    4. mental.

10. Adolescents who drink even small amounts of alcohol are at increased risk to: *(754)*
    1. develop acne.
    2. become obese.
    3. have a drop in their intelligence.
    4. have an accident.

11. Bulimia is described as: *(751)*
    1. binge eating followed by self-induced vomiting.
    2. resistance to eating due to fear of gaining weight.
    3. a systemic infection caused by a parasite.
    4. a secondary infection caused by a parasite.

12. A 16-year-old male who has broken off with his girlfriend threatens to kill himself. The nurse knows that this behavior: *(752, Nursing Tip; 753, Safety Alert)*
    1. is attention-seeking.
    2. should be taken seriously.
    3. should be ignored.
    4. is a normal reaction to the situation.

13. What is the most appropriate nursing response to a parent who states, "I hope my son outgrows his ADHD"? *(749)*
    1. "There are medications that can cure ADHD."
    2. "The symptoms decrease as the child matures."
    3. "Does anyone else in your family have ADHD?"
    4. "These behaviors may continue into adulthood."

14. Children with ADHD: *(749)*
    1. may experience low self-esteem.
    2. are usually high achievers.
    3. usually have many friends.
    4. excel when given tasks that require intricate work.

15. An adolescent tells the nurse he has needed to increase his alcohol intake to feel its effect. The nurse recognizes that which situation has developed? *(754)*
    1. Psychological dependence
    2. Physical dependence
    3. Tolerance to the substance
    4. Withdrawal symptoms

CASE STUDY

1. Nine-year-old Christopher has arrived at the same-day surgery unit for dental extractions. Christopher was diagnosed with autism when he was 3 years old.
   a. What factors might influence Christopher's reaction to this hospital experience?
   b. You will be admitting Christopher to the unit. What information specific to autism should you elicit from Christopher's mother during the admission process?
   c. His mother tells you that Christopher is very anxious about his surgery. What strategies will you use to interact with him?
   d. After Christopher has been taken to the operating room, his mother says, "I don't understand why my other children seem to resent Christopher." What do you think is the reason for this? How would you respond to this statement?

THINKING CRITICALLY

1. In what way should care be altered when caring for a child with asthma who is also diagnosed as having ADHD?

APPLYING KNOWLEDGE

1. List two nursing diagnoses associated with depression. Discuss in a group how nursing care should be implemented for these diagnoses.

2. Care for a child with an emotional disorder who is admitted to the hospital for a physical problem.

3. Interview the family members of a child with ADHD. What impact has this condition had on them, individually and as a family?

Complementary and Alternative Therapies in Maternity and Pediatric Nursing

chapter

34

Answer Key: A complete answer key can be found on the Student Evolve website.

LEARNING ACTIVITIES

1. Give examples of the following therapies. Can you identify examples other than those listed in the text? *(760)*

    a. Complementary therapy: _____

    _____

    b. Alternative therapy: _____

    _____

2. What is the current status of regulation and licensure in the United States related to CAM therapies? *(760-761)*

    _____

    _____

    _____

    _____

3. a. What conditions can massage therapy benefit? *(763)* _____

    _____

    b. What are contraindications for use of massage therapy? Why? *(763)* _____

    _____

    _____

4. a. What is the use of a wristband that uses transcutaneous electrical nerve stimulation (TENS) during pregnancy? *(763)* _____

    _____

    b. What acupoints should be avoided during pregnancy and why? *(765)* _____

    _____

    _____

5. What are cautions and potential risks of homeopathic medicines? *(765)* _____

_____

_____

6. a. List some essential oils that should not be used during pregnancy aromatherapy. *(765)* _____

_____

_____

b. List essential oils that may be beneficial during pregnancy. What are their effects? *(765)* _____

_____

_____

c. List essential oils that may benefit children with chronic pain. *(765, Nursing Tip)* _____

_____

_____

7. a. How is guided imagery believed to be therapeutic? *(765)* _____

_____

b. How can a nurse use guided imagery to help a woman in labor? *(765)* _____

_____

_____

8. What are the cautions if the following people use herbal remedies? *(766-767)*

a. Pregnant women: _____

_____

b. Breastfeeding women: _____

_____

c. Children: _____

_____

9. List 11 herbs that promote menstruation and may cause miscarriage. *(767; Box 34-2)*

   a. _____

   b. _____

   c. _____

   d. _____

   e. _____

   f. _____

   g. _____

   h. _____

   i. _____

   j. _____

   k. _____

10. List four methods used as an alternative to hormone replacement therapy to manage the discomforts of menopause. *(767, 769; Table 34-4)*

   a. _____

   b. _____

   c. _____

   d. _____

REVIEW QUESTIONS

1. What is the most important reason a nurse should ask specifically about use of complementary or alternative therapy when admitting a patient to the hospital? *(761-762)*
   1. Use of these therapies gives insight into the person's cultural background.
   2. Most therapies are promoted by those with little education in their use.
   3. Knowledge of possible interactions with prescribed drugs reduces the chance of complications.
   4. The patient and family should be educated about the harmful effects of most complementary therapies.

2. A woman is troubled by hot flashes as she approaches menopause. She wants to avoid hormone replacement therapy because her mother had breast cancer and asks the nurse if natural remedies will help her. The best nursing response is that: *(767, 769)*
   1. these discomforts are normal for menopause and will gradually go away as she ages.
   2. some herbs may help her symptoms but she should consult her physician before using them.
   3. most herbs are regulated by the Food and Drug Administration as estrogen would be regulated.
   4. heat therapy is the most reliable way to reduce nighttime hot flashes.

3. A 3-year-old child is hospitalized for pneumonia. The nurse notes marks on the abdomen and asks the parents about how the child received them. The parents reply that they often use "coin rubbing" when the child is ill. Based on this explanation, the nurse should: *(763; Fig. 34-2)*
   1. document the marks and the parents' explanation for them.
   2. consult with child protective services because of possible abuse.
   3. explain to the parents that this practice cannot heal an infection.
   4. tell the parents that coin rubbing is dangerous to small children.

4. Energy therapy that may relieve nausea and vomiting associated with chemotherapy is: *(763)*
   1. effleurage of the abdomen.
   2. cold applied to the head.
   3. aromatherapy with essential oils and essences.
   4. transcutaneous electrical nerve stimulation.

5. A woman comes to clinic for her regular prenatal visit. She tells the nurse that acupressure has helped her with many discomforts, including the nausea she felt during early pregnancy. The best nursing response is to explain that: *(765)*
   1. acupressure on the bottom of her foot can help relieve the backache that often occurs during late pregnancy.
   2. acupuncture is safer than acupressure for relief of discomforts that are common during early and late pregnancy.
   3. several areas for pressure should be avoided during pregnancy to reduce the risk for preterm birth.
   4. it is best to avoid all types of unproven complementary therapies when she is pregnant.

6. When determining the dose of herbal therapy, the practitioner uses the: *(766)*
   1. person's body weight.
   2. person's age and sex.
   3. largest dose the person can tolerate.
   4. immune status of the person.

7. A woman has taken a number of vitamins and herbal therapies throughout her pregnancy. To avoid infection while she is breastfeeding she takes large quantities of vitamin C. The nurse should advise the woman that: *(767)*
   1. high-dose vitamin C can reduce the chance of infection in both her and the baby.
   2. vitamin C is a fat-soluble vitamin and should not be taken in large doses.
   3. taking vitamin C with a milk product will enhance its absorption.
   4. colic is more likely in the baby if she takes large amounts of vitamin C.

8. A woman who is 30 weeks pregnant enjoys a sauna many times to help her relax after work. The nurse should advise her that: *(769)*
   1. it's important keep the heat level low enough to avoid sweating.
   2. all heat therapy is contraindicated during pregnancy.
   3. she should leave the sauna if her pulse reaches 120.
   4. she should have another person with her when she uses the sauna.

CROSSWORD PUZZLE

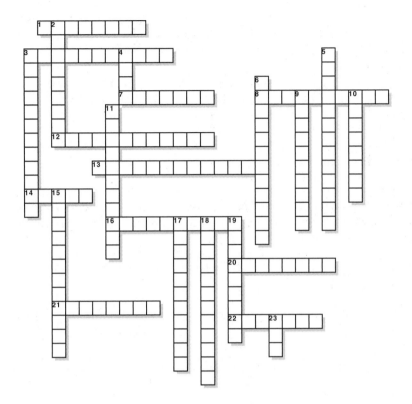

Across

1. Digitalis originates in this plant *(766)*
3. Unconventional therapy that replaces mainstream therapy *(760)*
7. Finger pressure used to prevent disease *(765)*
8. Use of plants, herbs, and earth minerals to stimulate the body's immune system or help specific health problems *(765)*
12. Therapy delivered by suggestions given to a person when he/she is in a state of induced sleep *(765)*
13. Type of massage to relieve muscle tension and trigger points of pain *(763)*
14. Opiate drugs are related to this plant *(766)*
16. Another name for traditional medicine *(763)*
20. Hindu healing that considers the biologic rhythms of nature *(765)*
21. Pathway to a specific organ or body part; used in acupuncture and acupressure *(764)*
22. Pressure, stretching, and manipulation of the fascia to increase muscle and bone function *(763)*

Down

2. Practitioner who combines traditional and manipulative therapy *(763)*
3. Use of concentrated essential oils combined with steam or baths to inhale or bathe the skin *(765)*
4. Acronym for electric current sent through the skin to stimulate nerves *(763)*
5. Nontraditional therapy used in conjunction with conventional therapy *(760)*
6. Therapy in which nerve energy is thought to restore or maintain health; care involves the relationship between the spinal column and nervous system *(765)*
9. Type of massage used during labor, often performed by the laboring woman *(763)*
10. Form of herbal remedy that contains a large quantity of alcohol *(766)*
11. Use of an electronic instrument to help a person recognize muscle tension *(765)*
15. Use of many medications *(762; Box 34-1)*
17. Stimulation of nerve cells using very thin needles *(764)*
18. Use of water to promote relaxation *(765)*
19. Mexican cultural folk healer *(761)*
23. Abbreviation for the agency that regulates drugs for effectiveness and safety *(762)*

CASE STUDY

1. Amy missed her period and thinks she may be pregnant. Her home pregnancy test is positive. This pregnancy is her fourth, although she miscarried two of the three previous babies. Her only child is now 2 years old. Amy is taking ginger for nausea. Use your text and other sources of valid information to determine the safety and effectiveness of ginger.
    a. List any reasons you find that ginger should not be used for early pregnancy nausea.
    b. What drugs did you find whose effectiveness may be affected by ginger?
    c. List all information sources that you use to reach your conclusions.

APPLYING KNOWLEDGE

1. Choose a complementary or alternative therapy that you have heard of, used, or considered using. Go to the website for the National Center for Complementary and Alternative Medicine at the National Institutes of Health at http://nccam.nih.gov/. Identify available information about the uses, effectiveness, and adverse effects of the therapy you have chosen.

2. Attend a childbirth class in which preparation for labor is covered. What complementary therapies do you see taught to expectant parents in the class?